100 Questions & Answers About Parkinson Disease

Abraham Lieberman, MD
with Marcia McCall

JONES AND BARTLETT PUBLISHERS

Sudbury, Massachusetts

BOSTON   TORONTO   LONDON   SINGAPORE

World Headquarters
Jones and Bartlett
Publishers
40 Tall Pine Drive
Sudbury, MA 01776
info@jbpub.com
www.jbpub.com

Jones and Bartlett
Publishers Canada
2406 Nikanna Road
Mississauga, ON L5C
2W6
CANADA

Jones and Bartlett
Publishers International
Barb House, Barb Mews
London W6 7PA
UK

Library of Congress Cataloging-in-Publication Data
Lieberman, A. N. (Abraham N.), 1938–
    100 questions & answers about Parkinson [sic] disease / Abraham
Lieberman, with Marcia McCall.
        p. cm.
Includes index.
Summary: A patient-oriented guide to the symptoms, diagnosis, and
treatment of Parkinson's disease.
    ISBN 0-7637-0433-4 (alk. paper)
    1. Parkinson's disease--Popular works. I. Title: One hundred
questions and answers about Parkinson's disease. II. McCall, Marcia.
III. Title.
    RC382.L543 2003
    616.8'33--dc21

                                                    2002152130

The authors, editor, and publisher have made every effort to provide accurate information. However, they are not responsible for errors, omissions, or for any outcomes related to the use of the contents of this book and take no responsibility for the use of the products described. Treatments and side effects described in this book may not be applicable to all patients; likewise, some patients may require a dose or experience a side effect that is not described herein. The reader should confer with his or her own physician regarding specific treatments and side effects. Drugs and medical devices are discussed that may have limited availability or be controlled by the Food and Drug Administration (FDA) for use only in a research study or clinical trial. The drug information presented has been derived from reference sources, recently published data, and pharmaceutical research data. Research, clinical practice, and government regulations often change the accepted standard in this field. When consideration is being given to use of any drug in the clinical setting, the health care provider or reader is responsible for determining FDA status of the drug, reading the package insert, reviewing prescribing information for the most up-to-date recommendations on dose, precautions, and contraindications, and determining the appropriate usage for the product. This is especially important in the case of drugs that are new or seldom used.

Acquisitions Editor: Christopher Davis
Production Editor: Elizabeth Platt
Cover Design: Philip Regan
Manufacturing Buyer: Therese Bräuer
Composition: Northeast Compositors
Printing and Binding: Malloy Lithographing
Cover Printer: Malloy Lithographing

Printed in the United States of America
07 06 05 04 03   10 9 8 7 6 5 4 3 2 1

Contents

Contents

I can think of no one better to write this book. If anyone knows the questions on the minds of patients with Parkinson Disease, it is Dr. Lieberman. As Medical Director of the National Parkinson Foundation, he handles a program on the Foundation's website, *www.parkinson.org*, called "Ask the Doctor." Every day, Dr. Lieberman is asked dozens of questions, which he adroitly and clearly answers. So he is keenly aware of what are the issues that patients and their families want answers to. And he has set those questions and answers into this book.

This book will be a valuable resource. One could easily start at the beginning and go through it cover to cover. But is just as valuable to open it at random and read what is there to learn something new about Parkinson Disease. But the questions are organized along different topics, which is most valuable. The reader can quickly find the answer to a vexing question by searching for the topic in the Table of Contents and read about what is on his or her mind.

Dr. Lieberman has a gift of being able to communicate readily and with great facility. This ability comes across as one reads his answers to the questions posed in this book. This book is a marvelous addition to the literature on Parkinson disease and will be highly useful to those who want to learn what is on patients' minds and how to deal with these questions. Enjoy!

Stanley Fahn, MD
Scientific Director, Parkinson's Disease Foundation
Merritt Professor of Neurology
Columbia University
New York, New York

Who is Abraham Lieberman?

If you have Parkinson Disease, you may ask who I am, and why have the authority to write about the disease. I've studied PD for 30 years, and I'm currently the national medical director of The Parkinson Foundation, the largest charitable organization devoted to finding a cure for PD. The Parkinson Foundation (TPF) was formed in 2003 from the National Parkinson Foundation (NPF) headquartered in Miami and the Parkinson Disease Foundation (PDF) headquartered in New York. I am the Harold S. Diamond Professor of Neurology at the University of Miami.

My medical training is as follows: I'm a 1963 graduate of the New York University School of Medicine; Board Certified in neurology and psychiatry; and a Fellow of the American Academy of Neurology, the American Neurological Association, and the Movement Disorder Society. I trained in neurology at Bellevue Hospital, one of the largest and busiest hospitals in America, between 1964–1967. During the Vietnam War, I was a neurologist at the United States Air Force Hospital in Tachikawa, Japan, 1967–1969. From 1970 to 1989, I was, successively, an instructor, then an assistant professor, then an associate professor, and then a full professor of neurology at NYU. I was principal or co-principal investigator of more than 200 grants and studies of such diverse topics as Alzheimer disease, brain tumors, coma, epilepsy, migraine headaches, nerve and muscle disease, Parkinson disease, and stroke. Most of the studies involved inventing ways of evaluating these diseases. The studies were complemented by a large and varied neurology practice, seeing people from every corner of the globe who came to NYU to consult specialists in AIDS, cancer, cardiac surgery, endocrinology, GI disease, infectious disease, liver disease, neurosurgery, orthopedics, stroke, and psychiatry.

Beginning in 1970, but accelerating after 1980, my practice centered on Parkinson disease. This intensified during the nine years I spent as Chief of Movement Disorders at the Barrow Neurological Institute in Phoenix, Arizona, 1989–1998. Here I helped start the Muhammad Ali Parkinson Research Center.

My interest in Parkinson disease was stimulated by a revolutionary breakthrough, the introduction of levodopa, also known as L-dopa, by Dr. George Cotzias in 1967. The interest was sharpened by the presence at NYU of gifted scientists in biochemistry, neurochemistry, neuropharmacology, neurophysiology, and neuropsychology. I'm especially indebted to Dr. Menek Goldstein, a renowned neurochemist, and Dr. Albert Goodgold, a renowned clinician, who introduced me to the great thinkers in Parkinson disease and made me critical of myself.

With colleagues at NYU and the Barrow, I've authored or coauthored more than 200 articles published in major medical and neurology books and journals, including the *New England Journal of Medicine*, *The Lancet*, the *Journal of the American Medical Association*, *Annals of Internal Medicine*, *Annals of Neurology*, *Archives of Neurology*, *Neurology*, *Journal of Neurology, Neurosurgery, Psychiatry*, and the *Journal of Pharmacology and Therapeutics*.

In 1998 Mr. Nathan Slewett, Co-Chair of TPF, invited me to Miami. With Mr. Slewett's encouragement and support, I started a major Parkinson disease website: *www.Parkinson.org*. The site receives more than 100,000 "hits" a day and more than 100 questions a day from 25,000 people with PD from every corner of the world: from Algeria to Australia, from Alberta to Argentina.

On a personal note, I've been married 37 years to Ina Lieberman, a pediatric anesthesiologist. We have 4 children, two daughters-in-law, one son-in-law, and 3 grandchildren. At age 6, I had polio, spending 18 months in hospitals, clinics, and rehabilitation centers. So I know the anxiety, the uncertainty, the insecurity, the fear, and the panic centered around having disease—both as a neurologist and a patient. This dual perspective—patient's and doctor's—is central to the book you hold in your hands. *100 Questions & Answers About Parkinson Disease* is my second collaboration with Jones and Bartlett Publishers. Previously, I wrote *Shaking Up Parkinson Disease: Fighting Like a Tiger, Thinking Like a Fox* (2002). All royalties from both books will be given to TPF to support research toward finding a cure for PD. It is my hope that such a cure will come in our lifetime and make further books on Parkinson disease unnecessary.

Abraham Lieberman, MD
October 2002

The book is dedicated to Lynn Diamond and her mother, Selma Diamond. For 27 years, Lynn Diamond has been my patient, and she and Selma have both been my friends.

I met Lynn in 1975 when I was an unknown assistant professor of neurology at New York University (NYU). Lynn, recently diagnosed with PD, wanted another opinion. She called NYU, and they referred her to me. I, rightly or wrongly, was the designated local "guru." I don't remember my first meeting with Lynn—she reminded me that she "was the young lady who spoke softly, walked backward, and asked many questions."

Lynn was not self-important, nor flamboyant, nor intrusive, but, I realize in retrospect, she was observant. I had received a grant worth a great deal of money today, much more in 1975. The grant allowed me to hire a nurse, whose job was to ask why people did not take their drugs as directed. Was it because they did not understand instructions? Was it because they could not understand **any** instructions? Was it because of conflict at home? Was it because they couldn't afford to pay for the drugs?

Ruth, the nurse, spent 8 hours a day on the phone. We didn't learn anything we didn't already suspect, but Ruth gave comfort and support to many, many, people. When the grant ended, Ruth left. I could not afford a nurse whose sole job was to talk to people, no matter how comforting. During a visit, Lynn asked me what had happened to Ruth, and I told her. She said, "But so many people benefited. So many people were consoled. How much was she paid?" I told her.

Lynn, who had never availed herself of Ruth's services, was silent. Then she sat down and, in her small script, wrote out a check for Ruth's salary. Lynn had never struck me as wealthy; she had no "airs," she made no demands. How could she write such a check? Certainly I could not. And, for the next 12 years while I was at NYU, Lynn paid for a nurse—a nurse she never used, a nurse who was an angel to hundreds and hundreds of people with PD.

In 1982 I began to prescribe selegiline (Deprenyl). It hadn't been approved in the United States, and I had to navigate an extraordinary bureaucratic maze to obtain it, legally, from Hungary—at the time, a Communist country, part of Ronald Reagan's "Evil Empire." But I had to buy it. I bought it for 30 cents a pill (it's considerably higher now) and sold it at cost. One afternoon, I received a delivery while Lynn was in my office. She asked me about selegiline and how I got the drug. I told her. She nodded and asked, "Who pays for the drug?"

"I do," I said.

"And then you sell it?" she asked.

"Yes, but at cost," I replied.

"Suppose someone can't afford it?" she asked. I shrugged.

"How much is it?" she asked. I told her.

Lynn sat down, wrote a check, and said, "I don't want you to charge anyone for the drug." This, from someone who had no need for the drug.

When I moved to Arizona, Lynn and Selma Diamond gave the Barrow Neurological Institute a substantial grant to start a laboratory in molecular genetics. PD was not in their family, but they understood the value of genetic research and were prepared to fund it. When I moved to Miami, their generosity continued: They gave to the National Parkinson Foundation, to the University of Miami, to research, to education, and to all people with PD.

Lynn has had PD for almost 45% of her life. She has never been bitter, she has never complained, and she has felt the suffering of others. Twenty-seven years later, she is still, "The young lady who speaks softly, walks backward, and asks many questions."

I wish Lynn didn't have PD. But she does. I wish no one had PD. But they do. I can't prevent PD. Or cure it. I try, but I can't. Lynn and Selma can't prevent PD. Or cure it. But they try. I wish more people tried as hard and as unselfishly.

PART ONE

Some Basic Questions

What is Parkinson disease?

Isn't PD a disease of old people?

What causes PD?

More . . .

1. What is Parkinson disease?

Parkinson disease (PD) is a journey—a journey that, once started, will last a lifetime. Many people have taken this journey, have described the pitfalls, and have mapped the course. It is not a journey you will take alone: Your family, friends, and neighbors will come with you. You will meet many travelers along the way and will have several doctors who will serve as guides—to help you through the rough places, to point out the dangers, and to provide assurance and understanding. The many travelers who have taken this journey know it well and can tell you how they overcame the obstacles: Don't neglect them—listen to them! Although the journey is not a pleasure cruise, you can be comforted because you are not alone.

PD can start slowly, so slowly that it's scarcely noticed. A slight tremor in your hand—it could be stress, couldn't it? A twitch in your shoulder—it could be a muscle strain, couldn't it? Your spouse asks why you don't smile any more. Your children ask why you walk slowly. You ignore their comments, but in your heart you know they mean something. Things just don't feel right. Finally, you make an appointment with your doctor and are told that it could be PD.

Diabetes

a condition in which the body cannot process sugar, either because it lacks insulin or because the body has become resistant to insulin.

Dopamine

a chemical messenger in the brain; loss of dopamine is a key factor in PD.

"What is PD?" you ask. Is it an infection, like a virus? No, it's not an infection. It's a chronic condition, an imbalance like **diabetes**. In diabetes, you lack insulin. In PD, you lack a chemical: **dopamine**. Diabetes is a disease of the glands; PD is a disease of the brain. A lack of insulin results in a high blood sugar. Because a high blood sugar is easy to measure, diabetes is easy to recognize and easy to diagnose. A loss of dopamine in the brain is not easy to measure. PD is *not* diagnosed by a blood test, but rather by the symptoms that a loss of dopamine causes. The symptoms may include trembling of your hands, stiffness of your muscles, and a **movement disorder**.

Sometimes just your hand or your hand and your leg trembles, and sometimes your tongue and jaw tremble; rarely, your belly and chest tremble. If your hand trembles, your trembling stops when you stretch out your hand to pick up a cup of coffee and returns when you rest or relax your hand. This is called a **resting tremor**, a condition that differs from essential tremor, ET, a disorder sometimes confused with PD. The tremor of ET increase when you stretch your hand and stops when you rest it. The tremor of PD starts in one hand and, in time, involves the other hand. The tremor of ET starts in both hands at the same time.

The stiffness, or rigidity, of PD affects the muscles of your arm and leg; the stiffness is on the same side as the tremor. The stiffness of PD may feel like the stiffness of arthritis, but it is not associated with swelling. Unlike the stiffness of arthritis, the stiffness of PD does not go away when you relax your arm or leg; it's as though your muscles are always tight, always contracted.

The movement disorder consists of slowness of movement called **bradykinesia**, from the Latin words "brady," meaning slow and "kinesia," meaning movement. The movement disorder also consists of a hesitancy or an inability to start a movement (called "start hesitation"), and an inability to complete a movement (called "paucity of movement"). The movement disorder in PD may show up as a lack of movement—a lack of which you may not be aware. The lack of movement

Movement disorder

any of a number of conditions that affect a person's ability to move normally, or that cause abnormal, involuntary movements.

Resting tremor

a trembling of the hands or feet that occurs only when they are at rest.

Bradykinesia

a primary symptom of PD that consists of slow movement, an incompleteness of movement, a difficulty in initiating movement, and an arrest of ongoing movement are associated with this slowness. Bradykinesia is the most prominent and usually the most disabling symptom of PD.

Some Basic Questions

may show up as a "masked" or "poker" face, a failure to blink your eyes, a failure to swing one or both of your arms while walking.

Just as people age differently, PD affects people differently.

Just as people age differently, PD affects people differently. Some symptoms appear sooner in one person than another, may be more troubling in one person than another, or may not appear. Tremor, which everyone associates with PD, does not affect 30% of people with PD.

2. Isn't PD a disease of old people?

Although PD is more common in older people, it is not exclusive to them. The peak onset of PD is 60 years of age, hardly old these days; however, 15% of PD patients are younger than 50, and 10% are 40 years or younger.

For every person diagnosed with PD, at least two more have PD but have not been diagnosed.

There are about 1.2 million people with PD in North America, and because the development of symptoms is slow and insidious, the time between onset and diagnosis may be between 2 to 5 years (some say PD may start 10 years before it's diagnosed). Given the long latency between the onset of the disease (which is virtually unnoticeable) and the diagnosis, it is estimated that for every person diagnosed with PD, at least two more have PD but have not been diagnosed. About 50,000 people are diagnosed with PD each year. PD affects slightly more men than women (approximately 55 men to 45 women). PD occurs evenly across different occupational and socioeconomic groups, and the rate of incidence has not changed since doctors have been keeping records.

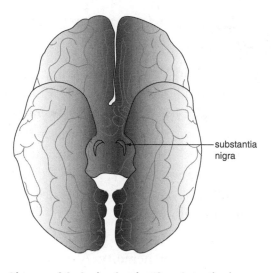

substantia
nigra

Figure 1   Diagram of the brain, showing the substantia nigra

3. What causes PD?

Parkinson disease results from a lack of dopamine in a region of the brain called the substantia nigra (Figure 1) The substantia nigra contains darkly pigmented cells (meaning "black substance" in Latin). It's not known why the substantia nigra is targeted or what targets it. At different times chemicals, dental amalgams, herbicides (such as Agent Orange), head trauma, industrial toxins, insecticides, pesticides, petroleum wastes (such as in the Gulf War), and well water have been implicated as a cause of PD. Although in an individual or a group of individuals one or more of these has been associated with PD, fewer than 3% of all people with PD have a cause that can be linked to the disease. PD is not infectious or contagious: spouses of people with PD are no more likely to have PD than spouses of people without PD.

Substantia nigra

a portion of the brain with darkly pigmented cells that is a principal location affected by PD.

4. If a relative and I have PD, does this mean PD is inherited?

Hereditary

passed down through the genes from parents to children.

Heredity or genetic predisposition may play a role. Between 15% and 25% of people with PD report that another relative also has PD. In about 1% of families in whom PD is known to occur in many members over several generations. Studies of the genetics of these families have identified specific, mutated **genes** that are linked to PD. However, the results cannot be generalized to all people with PD.

Genes

long strands of four molecules that determine the way in which proteins are made. Genes are the basis of heredity.

Chromosomes

collections of genes that compose DNA. All people have 23 pairs of chromosomes in every cell.

Genes are the basis for heredity. A gene consists of a long strand of four molecules arranged like beads on the 23 pairs of **chromosomes** found in each of us. Each chromosome carries thousands of genes, each gene consists of millions of molecules of the four chemicals that compose DNA. Genes determine the way in which proteins are made. If a gene is abnormal, the protein it determines will also be abnormal, and these abnormal proteins may cause PD. Scientists studying genetics have, so far, identified 3 mutations and 6 different locations in humans that are involved in PD. But there is much more to learn.

Free radicals

toxic molecules that arise from the breakdown and oxidation of foods and naturally occurring body chemicals.

One of the first genes associated with PD, which is on chromosome 6, was found by Japanese researchers and named the Parkin gene. The Parkin gene is found in the nucleus of cells and plays a role in "digesting" proteins. It appears that the role of the Parkin gene is to destroy defective or old proteins. If the Parkin gene is defective, the process of destruction is slowed—and the defective proteins increase, becoming toxic to the cell by oxidizing and releasing toxic **free radicals**. A second gene, called alpha synuclein, has been identified on chromosome 4 and is responsible for a relatively rare inherited form of PD. Alpha synuclein is found in **Lewy bodies**—small, iridescent pinkish spheres found in the dying nerve cells of people with PD. It appears that the gene mutation involved in production of alpha synuclein may start a biochemical cascade of events that eventually kills the cell. If the biochemical cascade leading to cell death, a process called apoptosis, can be interrupted by finding the right drug, a cure may be found. Researchers feel that an interplay between several genes and several environmental toxins may be responsible for PD.

Lewy bodies

small, iridescent pinkish spheres found in the dying nerve cells of people with PD.

5. Is Agent Orange or the Gulf War Syndrome a cause of PD?

Some studies show that people who work or live in rural, agricultural areas are more likely to develop PD than people who live in urban areas. Rural people are more likely to work with herbicides or pesticides. A few pesticides, such as one called rotenone, can cause PD in mice. At present it is not known if this is so in humans.

Agent Orange is the name of a herbicide developed for the military, primarily for use in Vietnam. The purpose of Agent Orange was to deny the enemy cover and concealment by defoliating trees, shrubs, and plants. Agent Orange is a 50–50 mix of two chemicals, known as TCDD. TCDD was mixed with kerosene or diesel fuel and dispersed by aircraft. An estimated 19 million gallons of Agent Orange were used in Vietnam, Laos, and Cambodia during the war. Early concerns about Agent Orange were that it was contaminated with dioxin. Dioxins are found in nature, and are cousins of certain chemicals that may cause cancer. In laboratory

Some Basic Questions

tests on animals, dioxin was shown to cause a variety of diseases, but not PD. TCDD is not found in nature, but is man-made. Questions have been raised as to the role of Agent Orange in PD. People who served in the military during the Vietnam War are now in the age range where PD most often occurs. At present it's not known whether the Vietnam War veterans who served in Vietnam, Laos, and Cambodia and were exposed to Agent Orange are at increased risk of PD. Nor do we know how much Agent Orange individual veterans were exposed to during the war. A sailor on a ship carrying sealed drums of Agent Orange did not have the same exposure as an infantry man moving, living, and fighting in the countryside sprayed by Agent Orange.

As many as 1 in 7 soldiers, sailors, airmen and women who served in the Persian Gulf during Operations Desert Shield and Desert Storm in 1990–1991 have complained of a number of symptoms referred to as the Gulf War Syndrome. Symptoms include memory loss, balance difficulty, sleep disturbances, depression, exhaustion, fatigue, and difficulty concentrating. Some physicians have concluded that Gulf War Syndrome doesn't exist—the symptoms the veterans complain of are related to a post-traumatic stress disorder. Other physicians have concluded there is a Gulf War Syndrome and that the symptoms were caused by a specific chemical, toxin, or virus the veterans encountered while serving in the Persian Gulf. If the symptoms are caused by contact with or exposure to a specific chemical, toxin, or virus, could such contact or exposure result in PD? In 1999 a study used a technique called Magnetic Resonance Spectroscopy to examine, in life, the chemical composition of the brains of veterans who served in the Gulf War. The veterans who suffered from the Gulf War Syndrome had lower levels of a specific chemical involved in energy metabolism. The lower levels of this chemical may indicate the loss of brain cells in the region targeted by PD. Although this does not prove a relationship between the Gulf War Syndrome and PD, many of these veterans are being followed to see if such a relationship develops.

6. Do viruses cause PD?

Viruses have been suspected as a cause of PD since the epidemic of **encephalitis lethargica**, the sleeping sickness that occurred early in the 20th century and was the basis for Oliver Sack's book *Awakenings*. In the winter of 1916–1917, a new illness suddenly appeared, and rapidly spread world-wide over the next 10 years. Symptoms of the sleeping sickness were so varied that no two patients ever presented exactly the same, and so strange as to call forth such diagnoses as epidemic delirium, epidemic schizophrenia, epidemic PD, and atypical poliomyelitis. Although there had been numerous smaller epidemics in the past, there had never been a worldwide epidemic on the scale of the one that started in 1916–1917. In the years that it raged, this epidemic affected 15 million people before it disappeared, as mysteriously as it had appeared. A third of those affected died. A third developed a disorder in which they would sit motionless and speechless all day, sleeping intermittently, and lacking energy. A third developed PD, but often not until many years after they had recovered from their infection. Why they developed such a "post-encephalitic PD" has never been explained.

Although no virus comparable to that of 1917–1927 has surfaced, some scientists believe PD could be

Encephalitis lethargica

the sleeping sickness that occurred early in the 20th century with symptoms resembling PD.

related to a virus, one that changes the genetic composition of the brain. Uncommon viruses such as Japanese B, eastern and western equine encephalitis, and St. Louis encephalitis have been linked to PD. In addition, such common viruses as the influenza virus (and possibly the West Nile virus) could be linked to PD.

7. Do drugs cause PD?

PD symptoms, but not PD, can be caused by drugs, but the PD symptoms are reversible upon stopping the drug. In contrast, true PD is an irreversible disease. Occasionally, a person with unrecognized PD is "unmasked" by the drug: the person's PD would have appeared, eventually, but it appeared sooner because of the drug. Drugs known to cause PD symptoms include haldol, prolixin, stellazine, and thorazine. Called major tranquillizers, these were the first drugs successfully used to treat the symptoms of psychosis and schizophrenia. Other drugs causing PD symptoms include orap, risperidal, and zyprexa. These are newer drugs and have been successfully used to treat the symptoms of obsessive compulsive disorder, psychosis, and schizophrenia. As a rule, they are less likely to cause PD symptoms than haldol, prolixin, stellazine, and thorazine. Not all medications that cause PD symptoms treat psychiatric problems: compazine and reglan, drugs used to treat nausea, vomiting, and acid reflux, may cause such symptoms. All the drugs have in common an ability to block fully or partly dopamine receptors in the brain. In effect, they cause PD symptoms by making the receptors unavailable to the brain's own dopamine.

Drugs known to cause PD symptoms also include reserpine (a drug used, at one time, to lower blood pressure) and tetrabenazine (a drug used to control dyskinesia, a condition described below). Reserpine and tetrabenazine deplete the brain of dopamine. This depletion is temporary, and levels return to normal after the drugs are stopped.

The incidence of PD symptoms in people taking these drugs varies from 15%–60% and depends on the drug, its dose, the time on the drug, the person's age (older people are more susceptible), and the person's sensitivity; some people are more likely to develop PD symptoms than others. Usually PD symptoms appear weeks or months after the drug is started (rarely sooner) and disappear weeks or months after the drug is stopped. The symptoms of drug caused PD are almost indistinguishable from PD. There are differences:

1. Drug-caused PD symptoms appear on both sides of the body at the same time. The symptoms of true PD appear first on one side of the body, and later on the other side.
2. The "pill-rolling" resting tremor of PD is less common in drug-caused PD symptoms (see Question 11). An action tremor, one that appears when the hands are moving and one faster than the pill-rolling tremor, is characteristic of drug-caused PD symptoms.

It's not known whether drug-caused PD symptoms are a "predictor" of the later development of PD. The PD symptoms may be associated with **dyskinesia**—dance-like involuntary movements. Dyskinesia may involve the face, the tongue, the head and neck, the trunk, the arms and legs. The movements are called tardive dyskinesia because they appear after the drug is started, or sometimes after the drug is stopped. Although drug-caused PD symptoms and tardive dyskinesia are probably mediated by different mechanisms, the two may

Dyskinesia

dance-like involuntary movements. Dyskinesia may involve the face, the tongue, the head and neck, the trunk, and the arms and legs.

coexist in the same person. This combination presents a challenge because the treatment of one may aggravate the other.

In another category are drugs that cause permanent PD symptoms. One such drug is MPTP, a narcotic-like drug, the actions of which were described by Dr. J. William Langston. The following passage is from his book, *The Case of the Frozen Addict* (Pantheon Books, 1995):

> George Carillo knew something was wrong the moment he injected the heroin. His arm burned as if hot lead were flowing into his veins, giving him a stunning high, the best he had had for years. Then he began to hallucinate strangely, trying to walk through doors that weren't there, hurting himself each time he plowed into a wall... The next morning George awoke feeling as if his body had turned to stone. His girlfriend Juanita was sleeping quietly on his shoulder, but when he tried to move his right arm he couldn't. It was stuck, wrapped around her body. Juanita pried herself free and helped George out of bed. Everything George did that day happened in slow motion—going to the bathroom, getting dressed, making breakfast. He had no desire to go out, but he had to show up in court or his parole would be revoked. Moving with glacial speed. George struggled... to get to the courthouse.
>
> The courthouse guard noticed a strange figure shuffling past the metal detector and assumed that he was intoxicated. George never made it through the door. He was arrested on the spot for being under the influence, a parole violation. Within hours he was in jail. Each day in his cell, George's stiffness got worse. By the fourth day he could hardly move his arms. By the sixth, he could not talk. He could see people and hear them, he could feel the sensation if someone jostled him. But he couldn't turn his head or reply if someone called his name. He was terrified.

Finally a doctor was called. Struck by George's appearance, he immediately sent him to the emergency room at the county hospital... The emergency room doctors were skeptical: Prisoners will try anything to get to a hospital, where the treatment and food (and the opportunities for escape) are much better. There was a good chance this patient was faking his bizarre condition. But there were other possibilities. Prison doctors sometimes give large doses of potent tranquilizers to chemically restrain agitated or violent patients. On the chance that George had been over-tranquilized, the emergency room staff took blood and urine samples. Since the results would take time, they injected 25 milligrams of Benadryl—a drug known to reverse their effects... But the Benadryl didn't work. Next, the physicians tried a stronger antidote, Cogentin, to overcome the effects of any tranquilizers George might have received. It had no effect. They returned him to the jail frozen and mute.

The next day both George and the tests came back. The tests were negative there were no traces of tranquilizer in his blood or urine. Not having any idea what they were dealing with... the physicians decided to push even harder to see if their immobile patient was faking his bizarre condition. First they scraped the soles of his feet to jolt him out of his state. No response... Finally, in exasperation, they tried smelling salts... They broke a capsule and held it up to George's nostrils, but again— no response...

Inside, George was consumed with anger. He could hear everything. He could feel everything... he had felt like throwing up when they passed the smelling salts under his nose. At one point he was so angry that he tried to hit one of the doctors. He willed his arm to move, and it did start, but it moved so slowly that nobody in the room noticed.

Satisfied that he wasn't a malingerer but having no idea what was wrong with him, the physicians sent George to the hospital... The neurologists had never seen a patient anything like George either... Trapped inside his body. George watched helplessly as the arguments flew back and forth. Maybe the heroin he had bought was to blame, but there was no way he could tell them. Various doctors came and went. They prodded him, pricked him with pins, banged him with reflex hammers, and shone lights in his eyes. After a few days... George was to be transferred to a special unit.

In the hospital George was diagnosed by Dr. Langston as having PD. Later, it was determined that George and several other addicts had developed PD as a result of injecting themselves with 'heroin' contaminated with a chemical called MPTP. MPTP was later shown by Dr. Langston (now at the California Parkinson Institute) and Dr. Stanley Burns (now at Southern Illinois University) to act as a "guided missile," specifically destroying nerve cells in the substantia nigra. The same nerve cells destroyed by the process that causes PD. The difference between MPTP-PD and PD is that in PD the dying cells contain a round structure called a Lewy body, but this is absent in MPTP-caused PD. The Lewy body is telling us something about what caused PD, but as yet we have not figured out what it is the Lewy body is telling us. MPTP has served as an excellent means of causing PD in animals. It has provided us with insights into how PD may start and progress. And it has helped in the development on new drugs for PD.

8. Do strokes cause PD?

Strokes are caused by blockage of arteries: the "pipes" through which blood flows. Arteries harden in older people, especially if they have diabetes, high blood pressure, high cholesterol, and if they smoked. If an artery closes, and if there are no arteries in the neighborhood that can replace it, the region of the brain the artery supplies is infracted: it dies. Unlike PD, where symptoms appear slowly and progress, in a stroke symptoms appear suddenly and do not progress. In PD symptoms do not go away, whereas in a stroke they may. Strokes do not cause PD, but occasionally a person may have many small strokes in the **corpus striatum**, the region of the brain to which fibers from the substantia nigra go. Strokes in the striatum may cause symptoms of PD. These symptoms do not respond well to PD drugs. The strokes can be seen on an MRI scan (magnetic resonance imaging). This is called "vascular PD." Sometimes strokes and PD coexist: having PD does not protect you from having strokes, and vice versa.

9. Can my job cause PD?

Two occupations have been associated with PD: boxing and welding.

Boxing and Head Injury

A small number of people, less than 1%, who sustain a significant head injury develop symptoms of PD. A "significant head injury" means the person was in coma for 24 hours or more, may have had surgery to remove a blood clot, and spent several weeks or months in a hospital. A minor head injury doesn't cause PD symptoms. A minor head injury is one that doesn't result in a loss of consciousness—or if it does, the loss of consciousness is brief. Such people are rarely hospitalized. However, there are people who develop PD who are certain their disease began after a minor head injury. For PD to begin, approximately 60% of the cells in the substantia nigra must be lost. These cells are not lost

In PD symptoms do not go away, whereas in a stroke they may.

Corpus striatum
a region of the brain named because of the large number of fibers that cross it—giving it a stripped or braided appearance (the name comes from the Latin "stripped-substance").

because of a minor injury. It's more likely PD was already present and the injury "unmasked" it. A problem arises when there's a lawsuit and a person claims a blow to his head caused his PD. The scientific evidence doesn't support this. How a judge and jury decide may be different.

Because of Muhammad Ali, the famous boxer who has PD, there's much interest in whether boxing causes PD. Boxing, when it causes brain damage, results in Alzheimer disease. This is not what Ali has: his mind is sharp. In several studies 15–40% of professional ex-boxers were found to have developed symptoms of Alzheimer disease. A few also had symptoms of PD. At one end of the spectrum is George Foreman, who fought longer than Ali but is on television doing a fine job selling his grill, with no obvious problems. At the other end are severely affected boxers, labeled "punch drunk." In between are boxers with varying degrees of speech difficulty, stiffness, unsteadiness, memory loss, and inappropriate behavior.

Symptoms, when they occur, usually begin shortly after the end of a boxer's career. On occasion they are first noticed after a hard bout. Symptoms develop an average of 16 years after they start to box, although sometimes they occur as early as 6 years after they start to box. Although symptoms are reported in amateurs, they are more common in professionals. They occur in all weight classes but are more frequent in heavyweights. The exact mechanism by which multiple and repeated blows to the head cause brain damage is not established, although it appears that the deep mid-line regions of the brain, including those involved in PD, are affected most severely. It is thought that heavy blows to the head results in microscopic damage to these regions. As the damage accumulates, minimal symptoms merge gradually into more obvious symptoms. The boxer usually is not aware of his difficulties; his wife and trainer are often the first to notice subtle personality changes. Confrontations with law enforcement authorities are often the result of lost social inhibitions or sudden changes in mood and behavior. These difficulties usually are explained away as symptoms of depression, anxiety, or even the enthusiasm of an immature aging athlete. An example of such behavior is the ex-heavyweight champion Mike Tyson.

Post-mortem examination of the brain of boxers reveal not the changes of PD—a loss of dopamine cells in the substantia nigra with the formation of Lewy bodies—but the loss of cells in several regions of the brain, mainly the frontal and temporal lobes but also the substantia nigra and the striatum. The changes resemble those of Alzheimer disease and include the appearance of "nerve fiber tangles" in the dying brain cells.

Welding

Metal poisoning can result from exposure to vapors or when metals are ingested in contaminated food or drink. Most metals are excreted through the kidney and feces. Some are also excreted through the saliva, the perspiration, and the lungs. After a metal is absorbed, its distribution depends upon its transformation, its binding to the body's proteins, and its entry into the brain. Welding is the process of joining metals together using a filler and an electric arc. The filler is a coated wire that contributes metal to the joint. The process of melting the metal and the filler produces fumes and gases that contain a number of elements, including manganese, lead, carbon monoxide, and fluorine. Welding may cause upper respiratory symptoms, pulmonary edema (water on the lung), pulmonary fibrosis (scarring of the lung) and lung cancer. Welding has also been associated with bladder and throat cancers. Neurologic complications include confusion and delusions from the fumes (called "fume fever"). PD symptoms have been described in welders. Although manganese miners are known to develop PD symptoms from inhalation of manganese dust, it's unclear whether this happens in welders. At Washington University in St. Louis, a study compared the features of PD in 15 career welders, to control groups with PD. Welders were exposed to a mean of 47,144 welding hours (5.4 years). Welders had a younger age at onset (46 years) of PD compared with controls (63 years). There was no difference in frequency of tremor, slowness of movement, rigidity, postural instability, family history, clinical depression, or dementia. All treated welders responded to levodopa. Motor fluctuations and dyskinesias occurred at a similar frequency in welders and the control groups. PET scans with 6-fluorodopa obtained in 2 of the welders showed findings typical of PD. This suggests, but does not prove, that welding causes a PD-like disorder. As postmortem studies have not been done on welders, it's not known if the pathology of PD in welders is similar to or different from PD in average people.

10. Can I die from PD?

In 1967, before levodopa, Mirapex, Requip, Permax, or Comtan became available, people diagnosed with PD lived, on average, 5 to 15 years from diagnosis to death. Death came in several ways.

1. People with PD became immobile and were confined to bed 5 to 15 years after diagnosis. Some developed difficulty swallowing. They gagged or choked on their food, even when fed carefully. The food was aspirated or swallowed into the lungs, causing pneumonia. The rigidity of PD restricted the movement of the chest wall muscles—the muscles necessary for inhaling and exhaling deeply and therefore necessary for overcoming pneumonia. As the pneumonia spread and the rigidity of the chest wall muscles restricted the body's ability to fight the pneumonia, it overwhelmed the body's defenses despite the use of antibiotics. Breathing became labored, oxygen levels fell, and the patients died. Sometimes the infection spread from the lungs to the blood, the heart, the liver, and the kidneys, so the patients died of sepsis (blood poisoning).

2. Patients became immobile and were confined to bed 5–15 years after diagnosis. Unless patients' were turned in bed every hour, unless they had skilled one-to-one nursing care, their skin broke down, and they developed pressure sores on their buttocks and on their lower back. The sores became infected and the patients died from the infection.

3. Patients became immobile and were confined to bed 5–15 years after diagnosis. Lying in bed, their legs rigid and immobile, they developed blood clots in their legs. The clots broke apart and spread to the lungs, shutting them down.

4. People with PD fell and fractured a hip, their pelvis, or their spine. This confined them to bed and, in turn, they developed the complications of being bed-bound.

*People diag-
nosed wit PD
now live on
average 15 to
20 years from
diagnosis to
death*

The introduction of medications such as L-dopa, Comtan, Mirapex, Requip, and Permax has changed the dynamics of this disease. People diagnosed with PD now live on average 15 to 25 years from diagnosis to death. The drugs postpone the day when people become confined to bed, and this, in turn, postpones the complications of being bed-bound. Antibiotics have improved. Skilled nursing care has improved. Air mattresses reduce the chances of bedsores developing. Special stockings can reduce blood clots from forming in the legs, and anticoagulants (blood thinners) can reduce the chances of blood clots breaking apart and traveling to the lungs. Do people die of PD? Technically, no. Death is postponed, but it's not prevented. But PD sets the body up for death. Whether patients die of PD, or of complications from PD, they die. The remedy is research to find the cause of PD or slow its progression so patients can enjoy more time with milder symptoms.

PART TWO

Tell Me More

What are the primary symptoms of PD?

What are some of the secondary symptoms?

I am seeing a neurologist. What should I expect?

More ...

11. What are the primary symptoms of PD?

There are four primary symptoms of PD. To diagnose PD, at least two primary symptoms must be present. **Tremor** is the most characteristic symptom of PD and is the first symptom in 75% of people with PD. It appears as a "beating" or oscillating movement, usually of the hands but occasionally of the feet or chin. The movement is regular (4–6 beats per second) and is rhythmic, with each movement resembling the other. The tremor usually appears when the muscles of the hands or feet are relaxed, when they're at rest. Hence, the name: resting tremor. The tremor usually, but not always, decreases or disappears when the muscles of the hands or feet contract during movement. The resting tremor of PD usually begins on one side of the body and later spreads to the other side of the body. The tremor usually looks like you are rolling a cigar, coin or pill between your thumb and index finger. Hence, the name "pill-rolling" tremor.

In 20% of people with PD, the tremor is also present, or only present, during movement. This is like the tremor in another condition often confused with PD: essential tremor (discussed in Question 13). Essential tremor, because it's driven in part by anxiety, may not respond as well to drugs for PD.

The rigidity of PD is described as stiffness or hardness of the muscles. Normally muscles contract and harden when they move, and relax or soften when they rest. In rigidity, the muscle of an affected limb stays hard and contracted. Stretching the limb is difficult. Because of

Tremor

involuntary trembling, usually of the hands or head.

rigidity you may not swing your arms when you walk. The mask-like or expressionless face that is characteristic of PD results, in part, from rigidity of your facial muscles. Many people with PD have "cogwheel rigidity," in which the arm or leg "catches" during movement, resembling the way a cog catches in a wheel. The small, illegible, compressed handwriting and the decreased eye blinking of people with PD are related, in part, to rigidity.

Bradykinesia means slow (brady) movement (kinesis). In addition to slow movement, bradykinesia also includes an incompleteness of movement, a difficulty in initiating movement, and an arrest of ongoing movement associated with this slowness. Bradykinesia is the most prominent and usually the most disabling symptom of PD. With bradykinesia, you may have difficulty walking and changing positions. The slowness and incompleteness of movement can also affect speaking and swallowing.

Postural instability is a lack of balance or unsteadiness while standing or changing positions. Often friends notice these changes before the person with PD does. If you are affected, you may have difficultly keeping your balance while turning or changing position. Some of the things that you did automatically, such as righting or correcting yourself after being bumped or pushed become difficult—and you may fall. The **postural reflexes**, which initiate these corrective movements, are located deep in the brain and may be affected in PD. Postural instability may not respond to PD drugs.

Postural instability
a lack of balance or unsteadiness while standing or changing positions.

Postural reflexes
reflexes that allow one to maintain balance.

12. What are some of the secondary symptoms?

Secondary symptoms are often combinations of one or more primary symptoms, or they occur less frequently and consistently than primary symptoms, or they are minor annoyances. However, some secondary symptoms can result in major discomfort and disability. Not everyone with PD even has the same symptoms—they vary from person to person. Understanding these symptoms can reduce their impact. There are several such symptoms, and although it's not possible to address them all, the most common ones are as follows.

- *Difficulty walking.* This is common in PD, and for many it is a major problem. Difficulty walking results from a combination of slowness of movement and postural instability. In PD your steps become shorter and shorter and you sometimes shuffle. Your arms no longer swing while you walk, and your turning may become slower and requires more effort. Sometimes you are involuntarily forced to take many tiny steps forward (called anteropulsion) before you can resume your normal stride. Sometimes you are involuntarily forced to take many tiny steps backward (called **retropulsion**) before you can resume your normal stride. Shuffling, anteropulsion, and retropulsion usually respond to levodopa or the dopamine agonists (Mirapex, Requip). In advanced PD, before starting to walk you may "freeze;" your feet seemingly becoming glued to the ground. Freezing comes on suddenly and can last for several seconds or minutes. Anxiety and frustration increases the freeze. Visual tricks and cues can sometimes help to restart walking; specialized walking sticks or canes can also help.

Retropulsion

begin involuntarily propelled backward when trying to walk forward.

- *Loss of smell.* This may be an early symptom of PD, usually appreciated in retrospect. This results from a loss of dopamine cells in a region of the brain called the olfactory cortex. Aromas of such familiar things as freshly brewing coffee or baking bread may not be noticed. A loss of the sense of smell can also affect the sense of taste, leading to decreased appetite and weight loss.
- *Micrographia.* A small, cramped handwriting results from a combination of slowness of movement and rigidity. Over the years, without your often being aware of it, your handwriting may become smaller and smaller and more and more cramped, sometimes becoming illegible. A business associate, a bank clerk, or your accountant may first notice a change in your handwriting.
- *Pain.* Pain in PD may take several forms. Sometimes it is a dull ache, a persistent nagging, or gnawing at a muscle. It is usually restricted to only one area at a time: a shoulder, an arm, calves of the legs, or the neck. In some people such pain in a shoulder or calf may be the first symptom of PD. Cramping in the leg muscles, especially at night, is a frequent complaint. This usually occurs after PD is diagnosed and is usually, but not always related, to a relative lack of dopamine in the brain: the cramping occurs as PD drugs "wear off." Headaches from rigid muscles in the neck may occur but are uncommon. If the pain responds to PD drugs, it is usually PD-related. But remember, people with PD can have pain for other reasons, the same ones as people without PD. When pain is severe and persistent, it must not be assumed it is related PD, and other causes must be sought. Some people with PD report a feeling of either heat or cold or numbness and tingling in their arms or legs. Sometimes, but not

always, this is relieved by PD drugs. Such symptoms may arise from a disorder of the autonomic nervous system (see Question 57).

- *Difficulty speaking.* Softness of voice (**hypophonia**) results from rigidity and slowness of movement of the muscles of the pharynx, larynx, and vocal cords, and the muscles of respiration (those that move air through the larynx and vocal cords). Hypophonia can vary from being an annoyance, forcing you to speak louder during ordinary conversation, to being a major problem in a lawyer or a politician. Hypophonia develops slowly, and you may be unaware your voice is inaudible. Hypophonia may be helped by a special type of training called the **Lee Silverman Voice Training** (LSVT). LSVT teaches you to strengthen your voice by singing loudly or shouting. LSVT resembles the voice training of an opera singer more than the speech training given to people who have had a stroke. Difficulty forming or pronouncing words is called **dysarthria**. Dysarthria is more common in people with PD-like disorders such as **Progressive Supranuclear Palsy** (PSP), Multiple System Atrophy (MSA), or vascular PD. Dysarthria results from rigidity and slowness of the lips, the tongue, and the throat.
- *Facial Masking.* Facial masking or **hypomimia** is a loss of facial expression resulting in a "poker" or "masked face" (as if a person is wearing a mask). Consequently, a person can't blink his eyes or smile, and always looks sad. The masking results from rigidity and slowness of the facial muscles, but it is often one of the first symptoms to improve with PD drugs.

Hypophonia

softness of voice stemming from rigidity in the muscles of the larynx and lungs.

Lee Silverman Voice Training

a method of training a person to strengthen his or her voice by singing loudly or shouting.

Dysarthria

difficulty forming or pronouncing words.

Progressive supranuclear palsy

a movement disorder with symptoms similar to PD.

Hypomimia

a mask-like expressionless face caused by rigidity of facial muscles.

Symptoms such drooling, bladder difficulty, constipation, impotence, difficulty sleeping, anxiety, depression, and dementia are discussed later (Questions 53, 54, and 92).

13. I am seeing a neurologist. What should I expect?

Although your primary care doctor may have recognized the symptoms of PD, he or she is trained in family medicine or internal medicine and may see few people with PD—perhaps 5 a year. Although he or she may recognize the symptoms, a family doctor may not have had the training in neurology to deal efficiently and effectively with PD. General practitioners may not be up to date on developments in PD, just as neurologists may not be up to date on developments in diabetes, heart disease, or cancer.

To have a diagnosis of PD confirmed, it is best to see a **neurologist**—better yet, a neurologist who specializes in PD called a movement disorder specialist (see Question 15). Most cities and towns have neurologists who treat mainly people with PD, who know about the complexities of PD, and who can adjust their treatment to you. The National Parkinson Foundation (NPF) and the American Parkinson Disease Association (APDA) maintain a list of "Centers of Excellence," neurologists all over North America who meet the standards of their organizations and who are qualified to treat PD. This list is available on their Internet page: *www.parkinson.org*.

It is important to find a neurologist with whom you can have a good working relationship. Treating PD requires more than an occasional visit. Like any chronic disease,

Neurologist
a physician specializing in diseases of the brain and nervous system.

To have a diagnosis of PD confirmed, it is best to see a neurologist.

it requires that you and your family work together with the doctor to find the best treatment or treatments. A knowledgeable neurologist can provide more than medicine to treat your symptoms: understanding, advice, and reassurance are important. If you have PD, a chronic **progressive disorder**, shopping around or changing doctors frequently is not in your best interest.

14. What does a neurologist do?

The neurologist will want to know why you came, your medical history, your family history (especially a history of PD or tremor), and what, if anything, in your social and work history may have contributed to your symptoms. Bring a summary of your medical history, including serious and chronic illness, hospitalizations, surgeries, allergies, medications taken, family and personal background, occupational risks, and lifestyle risks. If what you have to talk about is difficult to discuss, practice how to bring it up. If you expect bad news, bring someone supportive with you.

The doctor or his assistant may ask you about your activities of daily living. These include questions about your speech, salivation, swallowing, handwriting, cutting food and handling utensils, dressing, hygiene, turning in bed, falling, freezing, walking, tremor, and sensory symptoms. This review of your daily activities is not a laundry list. Careful and imaginative questioning is very helpful.

You should be asked whether there has been a change in your voice. Voice implies difficulty with the mechanical rather than the linguistic aspects of speech. An answer such as "yes, my voice seems to fade out at times and people are always asking me to speak up" is almost always diagnostic of PD. You should be asked whether you have recently noticed saliva escaping from

Progressive disorder

a condition that has progressively more severe symptoms over time.

the corner of your mouth. This is a private symptom often apparent only to you. The question usually elicits a reply such as "Yes, my pillow is wet at night, but I didn't mention it." Although drooling may be a relatively minor complaint, this symptom is associated with dementia in the minds of many patients and families (see Question 54). You should be reassured that your drooling does not mean you will "lose your mind." Prominent swallowing difficulty early in PD disease usually implies a PD-like disorder. Difficulty with handwriting, cutting food, handling utensils, dressing, and hygiene to some extent depends on whether your dominant hand is affected. If you appear to be unaware of any difficulty with these tasks, the doctor may ask you if you are slower in performing them. This question usually elicits a response such as "Yes, but that isn't anything, is it?"

It's helpful for the doctor to obtain specimens of your handwriting and compare them with past samples. This may show when your disease actually began. In some people it's reassuring to know they had PD for several years before they were aware of their symptoms. This implies their PD is progressing more slowly than they thought.

If your non-dominant hand is primarily affected, the questions should be directed to include those activities you usually performed with that hand. Thus if you're right-handed with left-sided PD, you may be asked how you button your shirt sleeves on your right side or how you wash your right shoulder.

People rarely associate difficulty with turning in bed with a disease, so they do not mention it and are surprised when asked. Such questions provide you with insight into the scope of your disease; you realize that symptoms as different as tremor, drooling, and difficulty turning in bed are part of the same process. During the question-and-answer time, the neurologist will observe your facial expression, your speech, your gestures, and your movements. The neurologist will observe you standing up, walking, and sitting. He or she will see how you rise from your chair and how you take your first step. Walking is a complex act, and a careful examination can provide many insights into your posture, the length of your stride, the way you move your feet, and how you turn. Because such observations require more space than is available in the neurologist's office, you may be asked to walk in the hallway outside.

The neurological examination has several parts. Rigidity is examined by testing muscle tone at your wrists, elbows, shoulders, and knees (and sometimes your hips) by holding the limb and moving it both slowly and rapidly. The testing of reflexes reveals much to a skilled examiner. Testing of strength or power provides more insight into how your nervous system works. Rapid movements are tested by asking you to tap your fingers to your thumb, to turn the palms of your hands up and down, to turn your wrists from side to side as though you're screwing in a light bulb, and to move your feet up and down as though you're walking. The examiner will be look at the amplitude, speed, and rhythm of your movements and compare your left with your right side. Tests of coordination are carried out by asking you to touch your finger to your nose and then to the tip of the examiner's finger. Another test involves running the heel of one foot up and down the shin of the opposite leg. This provides information on a region of your brain called the **cerebellum**. Eye

Cerebellum

the coordinating center in the brain.

movements and speech are also evaluated. The examiner may ask you to say "mama" or "papa" to test your lips. The examiner may ask you to say "Lulu" to test your tongue. The examiner may ask to say, "Ahh." This tests your pharynx. The sensory examination includes an evaluation of your ability to perceive a light touch, a pin prick, and your ability to tell (with your eyes closed) whether your thumb or great toe is being moved up or down. Testing for PD requires skill and practice on the part of the examiner.

15. How can I make my visit successful?

Your visit to your doctor is successful if, upon leaving the office, you know what's wrong and what the doctor can do to make you better. The visit is less satisfying, but still successful, if upon leaving you *don't* know what's wrong, but the doctor has told you, in words you can understand, *why* he or she doesn't know what's wrong—and can tell you what to do to determine the problem. The visit's a failure if you leave without knowing what's wrong, the doctor can't tell you what's wrong, and he also can't tell you how to determine the problem. It's also a failure if you leave more anxious, depressed, and confused than before. To minimize such failures, which are ever more common in an age of shorter visits, harried doctors, and more complicated problems, there are steps you can take. Start by asking yourself why you're seeing the doctor. If you can't say "why" in a few words, he might not be able to help. He's a doctor, not a mind reader, and he needs to hear *from you* what the problem is before he can try to address it.

When you visit your doctor, you're probably anxious or depressed, thinking "What's wrong? Is it bad? Will the doctor know? Can he help?" You may be angry (whether you realize it or not), thinking "Why me? Why do I have to be sick? Why do I have to see this doctor? And why do I have to pay for the privilege?"

Don't let your anger get the best of you. If after being diagnosed you don't agree with or like the diagnosis, don't "shoot the messenger." He may be wrong, in which case you're likely to resent the message all the more, but he may be right—and resenting the messenger doesn't change the message! And, sometime soon, you may need him. Remember, you're the one with the problem, not him—and you, not he, need help.

If you think you have PD, or your family doctor thinks you have PD and refers you to a specialist, you may wonder how to determine whether the specialist is any good. If your family doctor picked the specialist, it probably means that your doctor has worked with him or her before, knows the specialist's credentials and abilities, and knows how he deals with people. However, in an era where HMOs and insurance companies limit your choices, this may not be the case. Ask your family doctor or the specialist (or the specialist's office manager) the following questions:

1. *Is the specialist a neurologist?* To practice as a neurologist, a doctor, either an MD (medical doctor) or a DO (a doctor of osteopathy) must complete an accredited 3-year neurology training program.

2. *Is the neurologist board certified?* Upon completion of their training program, a neurologist takes first a written and then an oral examination in neurology and psychiatry. For a neurologist, 75% of the questions are on neurology and 25% are on psychiatry.

For a psychiatrist, 75% of the questions are on psychiatry and 25% are on neurology. Neurologists and psychiatrists, upon successful completion of their examination, are notified by the American Board of Psychiatry and Neurology as being certified in either neurology or psychiatry. Certification by the Board attests to, but doesn't guarantee, competence. Board certification (as evidenced by a diploma) is like a Good Housekeeping Seal. There are exceptions. The best neurologist I knew was not Board certified—he couldn't take the time to bother with the test.

3. *Is the neurologist a movement disorder specialist?* Within the field of neurology are accredited (by separate Boards) sub-specialties. *Movement Disorders* (which includes PD) is a sub-specialty but is not accredited by a separate Board. Movement disorders include PD (approximately 80% of the practice), the PD-like disorders (multiple system atrophy, progressive supranuclear palsy, corticobasilar degeneration, all described in Question 17), dystonia, essential tremor, Huntington disease, restless legs syndrome, tardive dyskinesia, and Wilson disease. To be called a movement disorder specialist a neurologist must take a 1–3 year fellowship in a movement disorder program after finishing his neurology training. Usually, the movement disorder specialist will display a certificate attesting to his completion of the fellowship. If you do not see such a certificate, ask where the specialist trained in movement disorders. There are excellent neurologists who treat PD but did not complete movement disorder fellowships. They, like all most movement disorder specialists, belong to the Movement Disorder Society (MDS). The MDS is an excellent organization, but it is not a guarantee of

competence in treating movement disorders. Any neurologist, or researcher can belong if they pay an annual fee.

4. *Is the movement disorder specialist famous? Is he or she a leader in the field?* Does his (or her) name come up when you search for PD articles on Google, Medline, the National Library of Medicine, or Scirus.com? Is he or she listed in the "Best Doctors in America" guide? Is he or she on television whenever there's a "breaking" story on PD? Is he or she Michael J. Fox's, Janet Reno's, or the Pope's doctor? The above reveals the specialist is familiar with PD and its nuances—but he or she *still* may not be right for you. He or she may be too busy doing research, writing articles, giving speeches, or traveling to see you when you want to be seen. Or, when you do get an appointment, you may only be able to see one of his fellows or associates. And while he may be available for Michael J. Fox, Janet Reno, or the Pope, he may not be available for you.

As you look for a neurologist that's right for you, you'll probably have many questions. Although you're anxious, afraid, depressed, and you may not remember everything you want to ask, try not to come with a long list. List the 3 or 4 main problems, complaints, or concerns in their order of importance to you. If you're satisfied the doctor has answered your 3 or 4 main problems, complaints, or concerns, and there are others you want the doctor (and not his staff) to answer, make a return appointment.

If you're going to see the doctor because you think you have PD, say exactly what prompted you to come. The following are examples: "I think I have PD because I have a tremor." "My wife [or a friend or another doctor] thinks I might have PD." "I saw Muhammad Ali, or Michael J. Fox, or Janet Reno, or the Pope on television, and I think I have what they have."

On your first visit, take a family member or friend. They will provide you with emotional support and comfort. They're also more likely to be objective and to hear what the specialist said rather than what you thought he said. A word of caution: Too many family members or friends in the room (more than two) changes the nature of the visit. If you have small children, get a babysitter: children may be frightened by being in a doctor's office, and they can cry and be disruptive.

Look for a courteous, caring, and polite staff, a clean office, and information on PD: books, pamphlets, and newsletters. Look for nurse or an assistant who asks you to fill out a form regarding PD. Such forms tell the specialist what he thinks is important. The questions asked, the clarity with which they are asked, and the detail they include will give you an idea as to how the specialist thinks. Waits of more than half an hour are rarely justified. Before you visit, ask whether the doctor goes to the hospital before seeing patients. If he does, this may result in delays because of unforeseen emergencies. If the doctor goes to the hospital, ask for an appointment on a day he does not go. If you asked the doctor to "squeeze you in," and he did, expect a delay. A doctor who will see you as an emergency or as a favor will generally set a time he can see you, or he will say, "I cannot fit you in, but I can have my associate or my colleague do so."

Although the diagnosis of PD may be apparent as soon as you walk in, the doctor should stifle the urge to make a quick diagnosis. To begin with, the diagnosis may be incorrect or, if correct, such a quick diagnosis can be

On your first visit, take a family member or friend.

Tell Me More

disturbing and not appreciated by you or your family. At the beginning of the illness, you and your family are frightened and anxious. You have probably sensed something is wrong but have denied or dismissed the symptoms. Now you and your family are feeling guilty and angry for not seeking help sooner. If a stranger, even the doctor, rapidly points out the obvious, it succeeds only in reinforcing your guilt and redirecting the anger toward the doctor. A recurrent theme of patients seeking another opinion is that the previous doctor "didn't examine me or listen to me." For a satisfactory doctor-patient relationship to be established, the doctor must appear caring and involved. After such a relationship has been established, his diagnosis is more likely to be accepted and his recommendations followed.

During the history, you may make a remark that confirms the diagnosis. Statements such as the following are almost diagnostic of PD: "My hand only begins to shake when I sit down" or "My handwriting has gotten so small that the bank won't cash my checks." It may become apparent to the doctor that you are not aware of any difficulty either because of denial or because of your inability to sense the difficulty. Although tremor and difficulty moving are prominent symptoms in PD, there may also be perceptual, behavioral, and personality changes that can interfere with your ability to recognize your difficulties. It may also become apparent during the examination that there is marital discord. A spouse who constantly answers for you without being asked or remarks that you "walk bent down like an ape" will not be the sympathetic caregiver necessary for successful management. Marital discord should be addressed. This is best done in a subsequent visit after the doctor has a better understanding of your family dynamics. It's helpful if the doctor asks whether any family member or friend has PD.

The diagnosis of PD is made after taking a history and by performing an examination in the office. A movement disorder specialist should be able to diagnose PD and be correct 85% of the time. Sometimes, because of unusual symptoms or because of an unusual finding during the examination the doctor may order an MRI scan. An MRI scan does not diagnose PD, but it can rule out other conditions that may mimic PD. Rarely, a PET or a SPECT scan using a special isotope may be necessary to confirm the diagnosis.

16. Are there tests for PD?

No specific test is currently available to determine whether PD is the cause of your symptoms. A disease-specific **biological marker** for PD has not been found. The only conclusive test for PD is a postmortem examination of the brain. Taking a history of your symptoms, their relationship to one another, their evolution, and performing a neurological examination is, at present, the best way of making a diagnosis. **Magnetic resonance imaging** (MRI) will not make a diagnosis of PD. It may reveal disorders such as multiple strokes, hydrocephalus (a fluid build-up in the brain) or a tumor that can mimic the symptoms of PD. PET and SPECT scans are relatively new and have provided much heretofore unavailable information about the state of the substantia nigra in living people. However, they are not readily available and require experts to interpret them. In time, PET and SPECT scans may become major adjuncts to the neurological examination.

Biological marker

a specific protein or genetic change that distinguishes a particular disease or condition.

Magnetic resonance imaging (MRI)

a technique that creates 3-dimensional images of body structures using strong magnetic fields.

17. Do these symptoms mean PD? Can they mean something else?

The symptoms of PD are called **parkinsonism**, but not all people with parkinsonism have PD. In fact, some of the symptoms of PD may be present in other diseases, the pathology and causes of which are different from PD. These PD-like disorders initially may be difficulty to distinguish from PD. In time, over several years, the differences become apparent. Occasionally, when doubt persists, a trial of levodopa may be given. Improvement occurs in PD; improvement is less consistent, or not present in the PD-like disorders (Figure 2). Magnetic resonance imaging (MRI) is not helpful in diagnosing PD, the PD-like disorders, or in distinguishing PD from the PD-like disorders. **Positron emission tomography** (PET scans) or single photon

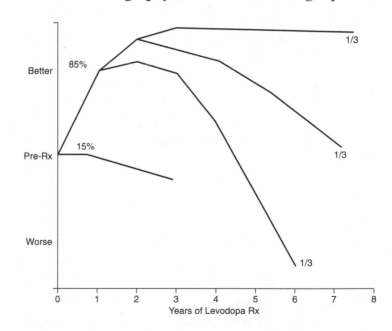

Figure 2   Curves showing how levodopa therapy affects PD patients over time, with 85% of patients having an improvement of symptoms in the first two years. Over time, about 1/3 of these responsive patients show a marked decline, 1/3 return to near pre-treatment levels, and 1/3 remain consistently better with levodopa.

emission computed tomography (SPECT scans) using specialized isotopes are increasingly being used to diagnose PD and distinguish PD from the PD-like disorders. However, these tests are not widely available and require expert interpretation.

The PD-like disorders can be divided into two classes to simplify their understanding. The first class is the **akinetic-rigid syndromes**, which are marked by stiffness and a lack of movement. The second are marked by excessive movement, called **hyperkinetic syndromes**.

Progressive supranuclear palsy (PSP) is the most common of the akinetic-rigid disorders. For every 100 people with PD, there are 5 with PSP. In addition to the main symptoms of PD—rigidity, bradykinesia, and postural instability—people with PSP become unable to move their eyes. People with PSP usually have major problems with balance, so they fall frequently. Unlike PD, falling is usually an early and not a late symptom. PSP, unlike PD, begins on both sides at the same time, occurs without tremor, and responds poorly or not at all to drugs. PSP progresses more rapidly than PD. On post-mortem examination PSP looks different from PD.

Multiple-system atrophy (MSA) may mimic PD, but usually occurs without tremor, responds poorly or not at all to drugs, and progresses more rapidly than PD. MSA has three subgroups: (1) The Shy-Drager variant resembles PD but is dominated by autonomic nervous system symptoms, such as drops in blood pressure on standing, bladder and bowel problems, and impotence. (2) The Striato-nigral variant (abbreviated SND) resembles PD but does not respond to PD drugs.

Akinetic-rigid syndromes
movement disorders marked by stiffness and a lack of movement.

Hyperkinetic
excessive movement.

(3) The olivo-ponto-cerebellar atrophy variant (OPCA) is dominated by difficulty with walking and balance, called **ataxia**. Falls are not as frequent as in the balance difficulty of PSP. On post-mortem examination MSA looks different from PSP and PD.

Corticobasilar degeneration (CBD) resembles PSP. Unlike PSP, which starts on both sides simultaneously, CBD may start first on one side. Rigidity is more of a problem than in PSP. Unlike PSP, in which eye movements are always affected, in CBD eye movement may not be affected. Falls are frequent in both CBD and PSP. For every 100 people with PD, 1 has CBD. On post-mortem examination CBD resembles PSP but looks different from PD and MSA.

Essential tremor (ET), a hyper-kinetic disorder, is the most common movement disorder. ET is 10–20 times more common than PD. However, in fewer than 2% the tremor of ET sufficiently is disabling to require treatment. ET affects primarily the hands, less often the head, and rarely the feet. ET, unlike PD, starts in both hands simultaneously. The tremor of ET, unlike the tremor of PD, appears when the hands are moving. The tremor of ET can be disabling, affecting fine motor skills such as shaving, buttoning your clothes, or feeding yourself. In ET, the handwriting becomes shaky, but it does not become small or cramped as in PD. Alcohol helps ET; an occasional drink may work wonders. Alcohol is less beneficial in PD. The affects of alcohol on ET are not well understood, and the overuse of alcohol could, of course, lead to dependence. In general, the drugs for PD do not help ET. ET responds to drugs such as mysoline (a drug used to treat epilepsy),

Ataxia
difficulty with walking and balancing.

Corticobasilar degeneration
a movement disorder that resembles PD but does not respond to PD drugs.

inderal (a drug used to treat high blood pressure), and benzodiazepines (drugs used to treat anxiety). Anxiety increases the tremor of ET and PD.

18. I have PD. What do I do?

If you have been diagnosed with PD, you may feel many conflicting emotions. You may fear becoming physically, emotionally, and economically dependent on others, or you may worry because the money that you've saved for retirement may have to go toward paying medical expenses. You may think that you no longer control your future or that you're alone and isolated. All of these concerns are normal; however, there are things you can and should do to take control of PD.

Your first reaction may be denial. You may wonder whether you heard the diagnosis right or if it is correct. Such a reaction gives you time to digest the news and formulate a response. "Nobody in my family has it," you say. "I'm sure it's stress. If I rearrange my schedule, exercise regularly, pay attention to what I eat, and get a good night of sleep, my symptoms will go away." Although exercise, nutrition, stress management, and rest are important, they won't cure PD. Your first reaction may also be relief that your problem isn't a brain tumor or a stroke and that it's not your imagination, because you've known that something was wrong.

Your second reaction may be fear and anxiety. Realizing that you have PD can make you fearful and anxious. You and your family have no idea what to expect—thus, you think the worst. You may fear losing your job, your friends, and most of all, your independence. These are honest reasons for being fearful or anxious; however, an excellent way to master fear is to learn as much as you can about PD. Talk with people who have PD and who have gone through similar experiences. They can tell you what worked— or what didn't. Find resources, information, workshops, and support groups that can help you to understand PD. For example, the National Parkinson Foundation has more than 1,000 support groups throughout the United States and has an Internet page (www. parkinson.org) where you can ask questions about PD.

If fear and anxiety aren't recognized, they'll show up as hostility and resentment. You'll wonder what sin you have committed to deserve PD. Your anger will be directed at the people you love. You'll snap at minor slights or disappointments. If this happens, stop, think, and do the following:

1. Recognize that having PD does not excuse being angry with others. Facing the reasons for behavior is the beginning of self-awareness, and self-awareness is the first step in coping with, adjusting to, and eventually controlling PD.

2. Understand that loved ones are also upset because you have PD and are trying to be supportive, although they don't know how. Don't be afraid to tell them what you need. Don't be afraid to talk. Everyone will benefit.

Learn healthy ways to channel anger.

3. Learn healthy ways to channel anger. Talk honestly and frankly with your spouse, a friend, or a counselor. Start by connecting with the people around

you. For example, if you hesitate or "freeze" while walking, people may be puzzled. Rather than being angry, hostile, or resentful when they stare, say this: "I have PD, and occasionally I get stuck and can't move; it'll pass in a few minutes."

Your third response may be depression. Sadness, despair, and helplessness often follow anger and resentment, especially if unrecognized. These are symptoms of **depression**, which is common in PD. If you find yourself crying frequently, withdrawing from day-to-day activities, or sleeping too much or too little, you may be depressed. Seek help because treatments are available. A risk in accepting help for the physical aspects of your PD is that you'll become dependent on others. To lessen this, retain as much responsibility for yourself as you can. By doing as much as you can independently, you'll feel better about yourself.

Depression
chronic feelings of sadness, despair, and helplessness.

19. Why is PD called a movement disorder?

Movement disorder is the term given to a broad category of problems that includes disorders of increased and decreased movement. Movement disorders can involve all parts of the nervous system; the majority originate in the brain, although injuries or disorders of the spinal cord and peripheral nerves may also cause problems with movement. Diagnosing these disorders requires specialized training. Knowledge about the causes and mechanisms of movement disorders is growing rapidly, as are advances in treatment. Recent developments have added to the understanding of genetic abnormalities and are also revealing some of the causes of specific movement disorders. This expansion of knowledge has created a specialized field within neurology that is devoted to the diagnosis and treatment of these disorders.

Some movement disorders involve increased movement (hyperkinetic movement disorders). **Tics** and tremors fit this category. **Dystonia** consists of involuntary muscle spasms resulting in awkward and sustained postures (which may be painful). Dystonia can involve the eyes, neck, the trunk, and the limbs. **Myoclonus** consists of quick, jerking movements that can involve one finger or the entire body. **Ballismus** consists of a sudden flinging of an arm or a leg. **Chorea**, or dyskinesia, are dance-like, flowing movements of arms or legs, often involving every part of the body. Sometimes the disorders overlap. Movement disorders may arise from disease of the nervous system or from drugs. Stress or anxiety may aggravate all movement disorders. There are specific treatments for many of these disorders.

PD, PSP, and MSA, described in Question 17 earlier, fall into a category of disorders in which movement is either slowed or absent. Although the tremor in PD may resemble a hyperkinetic disorder, the fact that it occurs when the limb is at rest places it in the hypokinetic category.

20. PD is progressive. What does this mean?

PD is a slowly progressive disease, which means that the symptoms worsen with time. The earliest symptoms can be so subtle and vague as to be dismissed or taken for something else. When you and your family look back, you may see that the changes you thought were related to aging were actually part of PD. For

Tics

involuntary muscle twitches or movements.

Dystonia

involuntary muscle spasms resulting in awkward and sustained postures, which may be painful. Dystonia can involve the eyes, neck, the trunk, and the limbs.

Myoclonus

a movement disorder that consists of quick, jerking movements that can involve one finger or the entire body.

Ballismus

a movement disorder that consists of sudden flinging of an arm or a leg.

Chorea

movement disorders characterized by dance-like, flowing movements of arms or legs, often involving every part of the body. Also called dyskinesia.

example, the stooped posture of PD may be taken as bad posture, or the softening of the voice may be taken as hoarseness. When PD begins, usually only one side is affected, such as stiffness in a leg when you're walking or holding an arm flexed at your elbow and close to your body. As PD progresses, the other side becomes involved. Often you are not aware of the changes and don't think anything is wrong! It is your spouse or partner who insists there has been a change. Changes are not rapid in PD; in fact, if a change does appear suddenly, then it is time to check for something else.

21. If we don't know what causes PD, do we know how to cure it?

Not yet. Hopes are high for a breakthrough in science in the near future; researchers are working very hard to find both the causes and a cure. Stem cell research (see Question 72) is at the forefront and is seeking to isolate or transform cells from other sources to replace the dead and dying ones of PD patients. Researchers are also delving into the cause, or causes, looking at damaged cells and the processes that cause them and using the latest and best knowledge gleaned in human genetics.

Although science has not yet found the cause or the cure, it has continued to develop newer and better drugs to alleviate and manage the symptoms (see Questions 23-32). With a well-trained movement disorder doctor's proper insight, these medications can help PD patients control the symptoms and can slow the progression of PD enough that patients can continue to lead active lives and maintain their independence (see Questions 15 and 33-40). Surgery can also sometimes help to control some symptoms, but it cannot reverse the disease.

PART THREE

Treatment

What is the goal of treatment?

What drugs treat PD?

Why start with a dopamine agonist?

More ...

22. What is the goal of treatment?

Because there is no cure, the goal of treatment in PD, as in all incurable diseases, is to provide you with the best quality of life that is possible. Successful treatment starts by establishing good working relationships between you, your doctor, and your family. It requires working together to find not only the best drugs but also the best ways to live with PD. To accomplish this, it is important that you know as much as you can about PD and how your drugs work. It is not enough just to take your drugs. You must be willing to change your life to make the most of living with PD.

The goal of treatment in PD, as in all incurable diseases, is to provide you with the best quality of life that is possible.

23. What drugs treat PD?

Since its introduction in 1967, **L-dopa** or **levodopa** has been the most effective drug for treating PD. The cells in the substantia nigra take up levodopa and change it into dopamine. Dopamine is then transported along an extension of the nerve cell called the axon to the next nerve cell (Figure 3) in the striatum, where it interacts with specialized proteins called dopamine receptors. For a time, 2 to 5 years, levodopa may work so well that you may think you do not have PD—until you forget a dose or two and your symptoms return. Levodopa was the first drug to impact PD. However, levodopa has its drawbacks. The first is nausea, but when **carbidopa** is combined with levodopa (the combination is used in the drug Sinemet), the nausea is reduced. The second is that at higher doses, fluctuations (called **wearing off**) and dyskinesia appear. In wearing off, the effect of a single dose lasts a shorter and shorter time. The addition of entacapone (sold under the brand name Comtan), a drug that blocks an enzyme called COMT, helps by extending the duration of action of Sinemet. Comtan does not work

L-dopa

see *Levodopa*.

Levodopa

a drug used to treat PD that is transformed into dopamine by the nerve cells in the substantia nigra.

Carbidopa

a drug that is given with levodopa to reduce its side effects.

Wearing off

a condition in which medications for PD slowly become less effective over time.

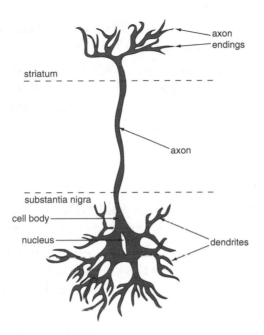

striatum

axon
endings

axon

substantia nigra

cell body

nucleus

dendrites

Figure 3   Dopamine nerve cell

Treatment

alone; one tablet of Comtan should be given with each dose of Sinemet. The side effects of Comtan are the side effects of Sinemet. If side effects occur, talk to your doctor about reducing the dose of Sinemet.

Wearing off or dyskinesia can be delayed by starting with drugs called dopamine agonists, which delay the need for levodopa. Dopamine antagonists, drugs such as haldol, stellazine, and thorazine, block dopamine receptors in the brain; hence their name—*antagonists.* Drugs such as **bromocriptine** (Parlodel), **pergolide** (Permax), **pramipexole** (Mirapex), and **ropinirole** (Requip) stimulate the dopamine receptors. Because their action is opposite that of the antagonists, they are called *agonists.* Whether you should start treatment with a dopamine agonist or Sinemet is a decision you and your doctor must make together. If you start on

Bromocriptine
a dopamine agonist.

Pergolide
a dopamine agonist.

Pramipexole
a dopamine agonist.

Ropinerole
a dopamine agonist.

Sinemet, your doctor can add an agonist later, and vice versa. Most people with PD eventually need Sinemet and a dopamine agonist. Mirapex and Requip are the most widely used agonists: They are easy to use, they are almost as effective as Sinemet, and, unlike Sinemet, they may slow the rate of progression of PD.

Selegiline, sometimes called deprenyl (Eldepryl), is a drug that blocks a specific enzyme called MAO-B. Selegiline, by itself, has a mild effect on PD. Selegiline combined with Sinemet may extend levodopa's duration of action (but less than when Comtan is combined with Sinemet). A newer drug, called rasagaline, also blocks MAO-B and may be more effective than selegiline. At one time it was thought that selegiline protected the dying dopamine cells.

Amantadine (Symmetrel) was developed, and is still used, as a drug to prevent the flu, influenza type "A." In 1967, a person with PD took amantadine to prevent the flu and found that her PD improved, so Dr. Robert Schwab in Boston tested amantadine in other people with PD. Now, amantadine helps about 50% of people with PD, but more than 50% of those whom it helps lose all or part of their benefit within a year. Amantadine has two mechanisms of action. It may release dopamine from the remaining cells in your brain. It may, in part, block the production of a chemical called **acetylcholine**, a chemical that acts to transmit nerve impulses in the brain, the peripheral nerves, the heart, the gut, the bladder, and the muscles. Drugs that block acetylcholine increase the activity of dopamine. Recently it has been discovered that amantadine, in some people with PD, decreases the dyskinesia caused by levodopa. The side effects of amantadine consist of a reddish violet discoloration of the legs called "livedo

---

Amantadine

a drug originally developed for flu symptoms that has been found to increase dopamine production and suppress acetylcholine in Parkinson patients.

Acetylcholine

a chemical that acts to transmit nerve impulses in the brain, the peripheral nerves, the heart, the gut, the bladder, and the muscles.

Drugs that block acetylcholine increase the activity of dopamine.

reticularis." This is usually accompanied by swelling. The discoloration and swelling disappear when amantadine is stopped. In older people, age 70 plus, amantadine, because of its anti-acetylcholine effect, may cause hallucinations. Acetylcholine, among other things, improves memory. Drugs that increase the production of acetylcholine in the brain, such as Aricept and Exelon, are used in people with Alzheimer disease and the dementia of PD because they improve memory. Hence, drugs that block acetylcholine may decrease memory or cause hallucinations. The side effects of amantadine stop when amantadine is stopped.

Before levodopa, the main treatment of PD involved the use of a class of drugs called **anticholinergics**. They are called anticholinergics because they block the actions of acetylcholine. Although all anticholinergic have partial activity in all the organs served by acetylcholine, many work better in one region than another. Thus atropine, an anticholinergic drug, is used to slow the heart rate; Detrol, another anticholinergic drug, is used to treat an overactive bladder; and drugs such as trihexyphenidyl (Artane) and benztropine (Cogentin) are used to treat PD. Artane and Cogentin are helpful in treating tremor and rigidity. They do not help bradykinesia. Anticholinergics are poorly tolerated in older patients and may cause side effects such as dry mouth, constipation, urinary retention, confusion and hallucinations.

Anticholinergics
drugs that block the activity of acetylcholine.

24. Why start with a dopamine agonist?

Dopamine agonists stimulate the dopamine receptors in the striatum directly, without having to be changed into dopamine. There are at least five types of dopamine receptors, labeled D–1, D–2, D–3, D–4, and D–5. The D–1 and D–2 receptors are important in PD. The D–3 receptors may be important in anxiety and depression. Sinemet works by being changed into dopamine, which stimulates both the D–1 and the D–2 receptors. This may be why it is so effective. The dopamine agonists, in contrast, stimulate different combinations of receptors. Mirapex and Requip stimulate the D–2 and D–3 receptors. This may be why they are less effective than Sinemet, but also why they do not cause dyskinesia—and it may also be why Mirapex has, in some people, an antidepressant effect. The agonists Mirapex and Requip have been shown to be so effective in treating people with early PD that the need for Sinemet may be delayed in many of them for several years. The risk of developing problems such as wearing off, **on-off**, dystonia, and dyskinesias are also lessened with the agonists than with Sinemet.

The levodopa in Sinemet has a short **half-life** of approximately 90 minutes. A half-life of a drug, like the half-life of a radioactive isotope, is a measure of the duration of the drug's action. A half-life of 90 minutes, or 1.5 hours, means that after 1.5 hours, the peak dose level of the drug has decreased by half or 50%. After another 1.5 hours, the dose level will have decreased by another 50%. Most drugs are eliminated from the body, and their effectiveness is gone, after 5 half-lives. The half-life gives you an idea as to how frequently you must take a drug to maintain effective circulating levels of the drug. Half-life is only part of the story, however. Drugs that enter the brain, such as levodopa and the dopamine agonists, are stored in the

On-off

in PD, the condition of alternating "on" (asymptomatic) periods with "off" periods in which symptoms such as freezing or dyskinesia are evident.

Half-life

a measure of the duration of the drug's action.

brain and may continue to have some activity, even when they have, on the basis of their half-lives, been eliminated from the body.

The short half-life of levodopa results in frequently alternating high and low blood levels of levodopa and presumably, high and low brain levels of first levodopa and then dopamine. This frequent alternation of high and low levels of dopamine is thought to lead to wearing off, on-off, dystonia and dyskinesia. It is as though you keep hitting the dopamine receptors with a "jackhammer" until you finally change their sensitivity. The longer half-life of dopamine agonists such as Mirapex (8–12 hours) and Requip (6 hours) prolongs the stimulation of the receptors and delaying the development of wearing off, on-off, dystonia, and dyskinesia. Treating young-onset PD patients with dopamine agonists alone can delay the onset of these effects. In people with more advanced PD who are already experiencing wearing off, on off, dystonia, and dyskinesia, adding an agonist, and reducing the dose of Sinemet, can decrease these effects.

Mirapex is usually started at a dose of 0.25 mg taken three times a day. The dose of Mirapex that is effective in most people is between 0.5 to 1.5 mg three times a day. This schedule can usually be reached in most people within 4 weeks. Requip is usually started at a dose of 0.25 mg three times a day. The dose of Requip that is effective in most people is between 2 to 8 mg three times a day. This schedule can usually be reached in most people within 6 weeks. Mirapex's main route of elimination is the kidneys. Requip's main route of elimination is the liver. Drugs that are eliminated through the liver are more likely to have a larger "spread" in their dosing level. In some people this is an advantage, in some not.

25. What are the side effects of agonists?

Nausea. Nausea is the most common side effect of the agonists and can be avoided or minimized by starting with a low dose and gradually building up as tolerance to nausea develops. Some people benefit from an anti-nausea drug such as Tigan. Tigan, unlike the anti-nausea drugs Compazine or Reglan, does not aggravate the symptoms of PD. By starting with a low dose of an agonist you are not as likely to experience as quick and as dramatic an improvement as on Sinemet. But by starting low, and going slowly, within several weeks substantial improvement will occur and you will maintain it longer.

Dizziness Upon Standing. Dizziness or lightheadedness upon standing usually indicate a drop in blood pressure. This is called postural or **orthostatic hypotension**. Postural or orthostatic hypotension may occur because you are dehydrated, diabetic, taking drugs to lower your blood pressure, taking diuretics ("water" pills), or have PD and are taking a dopamine agonist and/or Sinemet. Diabetes and PD affect the autonomic nervous system (see Question 57), the region that regulates the tone of your blood vessels—and by doing so regulating, in part, your blood pressure. If simple measures do not help this condition—such as sitting on the edge of the bed for a few minutes before standing up, taking your blood pressure drugs and your PD drugs at different times,

Orthostatic hypotension

a condition in which the body's blood pressure regulating mechanism fails to respond adequately to abrupt changes, e.g., when a person experiences dizziness upon standing up.

stopping your diuretic, and being certain to drink enough fluid to prevent dehydration—other medications may. The most commonly used drugs are Flurinef, a type of steroid that causes you to retain fluid, and Midodrine, which "tightens" the tone of your blood vessels.

Drowsiness. Periods of unexpected daytime drowsiness, sometimes accompanied by falling asleep, occur in people with PD who are not on any treatment as well as in people with PD who are taking Sinemet or an agonist. The periods of drowsiness may be more frequent in people who are taking an agonist. The periods of unexpected drowsiness, sometimes accompanied by falling asleep may be embarrassing, (especially if you fall asleep while a friend is talking to you), and, sometimes, may be dangerous, such as if they occur while you are driving. If you experience drowsiness while taking an agonist, do not drive until you have talked to your doctor. The periods of unexpected drowsiness usually disappear. Pro-vigil, a drug that promotes alertness, may help.

If you experience drowsiness while taking an agonist, do not drive until you have talked to your doctor.

Edema. Edema, or swelling of the legs, occurs in less than 5% of people on an agonist. It is usually mild. Rarely, however, it can be marked, will not respond to diuretics, and is a reason for stopping the agonist. A side effect that occurs with one agonist usually, but not always, occurs with the others. However, there are enough differences that if you have to stop one agonist because of a side effect, you may not have the same side effect on another agonist.

Another side effect, psychosis, is discussed in Question 27. Delusions, hallucinations, or compulsive behavior may be more common with agonists than with Sinemet in older people or in people "incubating" or harboring a dementia that was previously undiagnosed (see Question 55).

26. Do agonists slow the rate of progression of PD?

Two studies strongly suggest that this may be true. One study using pramipexole (Mirapex) recruited 82 newly diagnosed PD patients from 17 movement disorder clinics to participate in a 46-month study. The patients were randomly divided into two groups, one receiving Mirapex and the other Sinemet. They underwent SPECT using special markers to measure striatal uptake of dopamine at four different times during the study. The first was at baseline. The second was after 22 months. The third was after 34 months, and the final was after 46 months. A comparison of the treatment groups showed that patients initially treated with Mirapex had a lower reduction of striatal uptake than the group treated with levodopa (Figure 4). These data suggest that Mirapex does slow the loss of dopamine neurons. Figure 5 uses SPECT scans to show the loss of dopamine in the brain of people with PD versus people without PD. A similar figure can be drawn using PET scans instead of SPECT scans. Figure 4 also shows the loss of dopamine in the brain of people with PD treated with Mirapex is less than the loss of dopamine in the brain of people treated with Sinemet (levodopa). A similar figure can be drawn using PET scans instead of SPECT scans to show that the loss of dopamine in the brain of people treated with Requip is

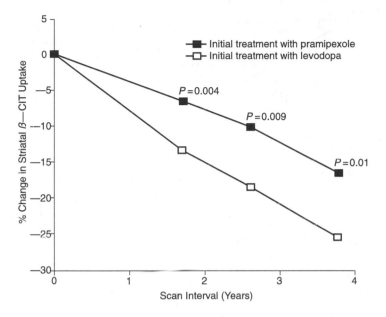

Figure 4   Comparison of striatal uptake of β-CIT in patients treated with either levodopa or Mirapex over 4 years

less than the loss of dopamine in the brain of people treated with Sinemet.

The second study involved 186 newly diagnosed PD patients for 2 years using PET at the beginning and end point of the study to visualize dopaminergic nerve terminals. These patients were evenly divided into two groups: One received ropinerole (Requip) and the other Sinemet (levodopa). Both PET and SPECT scans are able to produce accurate assessments of nigral-striatal dopamine content, although the PET scan study concentrated on a different region of the nigral-striatal dopamine system than the SPECT scan. The results of this study demonstrated that the Requip group had a lesser degree of progression than the Sinemet group.

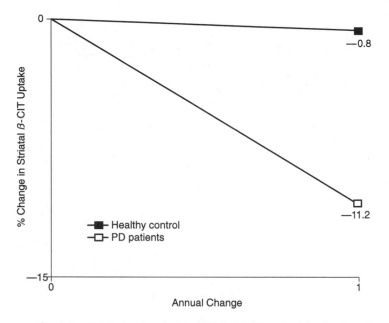

Figure 5   Graph showing the sharp decline in PD patients' striatal uptake of β-CIT, compared to a slight decline in normal people

27. Why should I take Sinemet?

Carbidopa/levodopa (Sinemet) helps reverse most of the symptoms of PD in most people but will not delay the rate of progression of PD. There are, however, concerns about how long the action of Sinemet will last. The levodopa in Sinemet is changed by cells in the substantia nigra into dopamine. As PD progresses, there is a continual loss of cells in the substantia nigra and the remaining cells become less efficient in changing levodopa to dopamine. There is no evidence that levodopa increases the rate of progression of PD, but as the cells die because of PD, the remaining cells are not as effective as they were originally. The early use of Sinemet, especially at doses of 600 mg a day or more of levodopa, is more likely to result in the appearance of changes such as wearing off and dyskinesia after 2 to 5 years. These are good reasons for starting with a dopamine agonist such as Mirapex or Requip and then adding Sinemet if the symptoms are not fully controlled by the agonist.

Sinemet comes in two forms: immediate or regular-release and a controlled or extended release, with varying doses of each, giving you and your doctor more possibilities to adjust the dosage for the most benefit. The dosage forms for regular Sinemet are 10/100, 25/100, and 25/250. The dosage forms for controlled or extended release Sinemet are 25/100 and 50/200. The first number stands for the amount of carbidopa in milligrams, the second number stands for the amount of levodopa in milligrams.

28. Why is carbidopa always given with levodopa?

When levodopa was first introduced, its major side effects were nausea and vomiting. In spite of its remarkable benefits, many patients could not or would not take it. The problem was in the conversion of L-dopa or levodopa to dopamine. The L-dopa or levodopa was changed in the stomach by an enzyme called dopa-decarboxylase (DDC) into dopamine. Dopamine in the stomach and circulating in the blood cannot cross the blood/brain barrier to reach the substantia nigra. However, dopamine in the stomach and circulating in the blood was reacting with the brain's trigger zone for nausea. To prevent the levodopa from being changed to dopamine outside the brain, carbidopa was added as a way to block the enzyme DDC. Carbidopa does not pass through the blood/brain barrier and insures that the conversion of levodopa to dopamine will take place in the substantia nigra, well past the nausea trigger zone. The addition of carbidopa prevents nausea and allows a smaller amount of levodopa to be used. Before the introduction of carbidopa the average dose of levodopa was 2000 to 4000 mg a day. With the addition of carbidopa the average dose of levodopa is 300 to 600 mg a day.

29. Why are there two kinds of Sinemet?

Carbidopa/levodopa, Sinemet, comes in two forms: immediate or regular release and controlled release. People with more advanced PD who had shorter responses to regular-release Sinemet were expected to benefit from the slower controlled-release form called Sinemet-CR. The coating surrounding Sinemet-CR slowed the absorption of levodopa into the bloodstream. It was thought this would overcome the wearing off effect that eventually appeared during treatment with regular-release Sinemet. Although Sinemet-CR is helpful, it did not live up to its expectations. In some people, because of their PD, their digestive system became slow, and the Sinemet-CR tablets remained for too long a period of time in their gut, never achieving high enough blood levels for maximum benefit. It takes approximately two hours for Sinemet-CR to take effect, and some patients did not achieve high enough blood levels for their Sinemet-CR to "kick in." Such people had to either be switched to regular-release Sinemet or their Sinemet-CR had to supplemented with regular-release Sinemet.

Dose schedules for regular-release Sinemet (25/100) are two to three times a day. In people with early PD, timing is usually not critical. Later, as PD advances, and the response to an individual dose of Sinemet shortens, people sense their Sinemet is wearing off or "turning off," so timing becomes important. To increase the effectiveness of regular-release Sinemet, it is important to take it approximately one hour before eating, as the protein in food can decrease the availability of the levodopa in Sinemet. However, Sinemet-CR may need to be taken with food to insure that it passes out of the stomach because little or no absorption takes place in the stomach.

30. What are the side effects of Sinemet?

Some of the "side effects" are not entirely side effects of Sinemet. Some (wearing off or on-off) result from progression of PD and the short duration of action of Sinemet; some (dystonia, "freezing") can be symptoms of PD (unrelated to drugs) or a side effect of Sinemet; some (dyskinesia) are side effects of Sinemet; and some (psychosis) are the effects of Sinemet and dopamine agonists temporarily "unmasking" an underlying dementia.

Wearing off. After an optimal peak effect from Sinemet is attained—the effect when Sinemet is working best, usually 1 to 2 hours after it is taken—it may be necessary to adjust the dose to prolong the duration of its effectiveness. When the effect of an individual dose of Sinemet diminishes noticeably between doses, this phenomenon is called wearing off. It is as though someone is slowly turning off a water faucet. There are ways to delay the onset of wearing off. The simplest being to give the next dose of Sinemet a little earlier, just before the effect of the last dose wears off. Sometimes using the sustained release form can add an hour

There are ways to delay the onset of wearing off.

61

or more to the time your Sinemet is working, the time you are "on." The addition of Comtan can prolong the time you are "on." The early use of a dopamine agonist such as Mirapex and Requip can delay the appearance of wearing off.

On-off. On-off, in contrast to wearing off, refers to the abrupt loss of efficacy of a dose of Sinemet, as though the dose, like a light switch, was suddenly turned off. On-off can occur with, follow, or be associated with wearing off. The "off" times, which by definition are abrupt, may last only a few minutes. Sometimes they are longer. Usually, but not always, they respond to additional regular-release Sinemet, but sometimes they persist—and can be as frustrating and as wrenching as a crashed computer program. The early use of dopamine agonists can delay or prevent the appearance of on-off.

Dyskinesia. Dyskinesia or chorea (from the Greek word meaning to dance) can appear as jerking, fidgeting, twisting, and turning movements. They may or may not be associated with dystonia. When dyskinesia and dystonia appear together it may be impossible to separate them. Dyskinesia occurs when a patient is over-medicated with Sinemet. Reducing the dose of Sinemet helps if the dyskinesia is not severe. But reducing the dose of Sinemet usually results in the person "turning off" and, to most people, being "off" is worse than being "on" and having dyskinesia. Adding a dopamine agonist such as Mirapex or Requip while slowly decreasing the dose of Sinemet usually, but not always, helps.

Dystonia. Dystonia are abnormal, slow involuntary spasms or cramps that can occur when the levels of levodopa are too "high" and sometimes, paradoxically, when they are too "low." Dystonia can appear as a sustained and painful cramping in your calf, foot, or toes, usually on the side most affected by PD. Less common are dystonia of the arms and hands. Dystonia can also consist of more prolonged, twisting muscle spasms involving your head, your neck, and your trunk. Some spasms may be related to wearing off of a dose of Sinemet, called "off" dystonia. These, the more common form of dystonia, improve when Sinemet or a dopamine agonist is added. Some spasms may be related to "turning on" of a dose of Sinemet, called "on" dystonia. Although dystonia is more common in people with PD who are treated with Sinemet, they may appear as an early symptom of PD, before any drugs are started. Dystonia may appear in disorders other than PD.

Freezing. Freezing refers to those times when it is impossible for you to start to walk or continue walking, as though your feet are "glued" to the ground. Freezing may occur early in PD. Such freezing responds to Sinemet or the dopamine agonists. Freezing may occur late in PD. And, although it resembles the freezing in early PD, it does not respond consistently to drugs. Indeed, sometimes it is made worse by drugs. Freezing may occur when you shift the position of your feet, when you change the direction in which you're walking, when you try to turn, or when you come to a curb, a step, or an open door. Almost anything that causes you to change the length of your stride, or even think about changing the length of your stride, can result in "freezing." It's as though a computer program, the one in your brain that allows you to easily and effortlessly change the length of your stride, suddenly crashes. Keep track of the time when freezing

Keep track of the time when freezing occurs.

occurs. If it happens when levodopa peaks in your blood, then reducing the dose may help. If it happens between doses of levodopa, then increasing the dose, shortening the time between doses, or adding an agonist may help. If freezing does not respond to changes in medication, a few "tricks" may "jiggle" your computer program and get you walking. As an example, if you can imagine yourself marching to a band or stepping over an object—be it someone else's foot or something imaginary—that may get you started again. The "tricks," in effect, restore the rhythm of your stride.

Psychosis. Hallucinations, delusions (believing things that don't exist are real) confusion, daytime drowsiness, nighttime insomnia, agitation, obsessions and compulsions—including obsessive interest in sex, eating, gambling, and shopping—occurs in people on PD drugs (see Question 55). The people are usually older, 70 plus years of age, and may be "incubating" a dementia. Amantadine, the anticholinergic drugs, selegiline, the dopamine agonists, and Sinemet, in that order, may "unmask" the underlying dementia. The psychosis may be decreased by stopping or decreasing some of the PD drugs or by adding antipsychosis drugs such as Clozaril, Geodon, or Seroquel. Unlike drugs such as Haldol, Stellazine, or Thorazine, these drugs do not aggravate the underlying PD.

31. I've been told that because I had a melanoma, I can't take Sinemet. Is this true?

Shortly after levodopa's release, the author of this book, Dr. Abraham Lieberman, saw a person with PD who developed a recurrence of his melanoma after 4 months of treatment with levodopa. Melanoma is a pigmented cancer of the skin. If not recognized and treated, it can metastasize (spread) almost everywhere in the body, which can be fatal. However, even if a melanoma is recognized and removed, years later it can reappear. Melanoma contains an enzyme, tyrosine oxidase, that can use levodopa as an energy source: hence the question of a relationship of melanoma to levodopa. After Dr. Lieberman's report, other doctors reported people in whom there appeared to be a relationship between starting levodopa or Sinemet and recurrence of melanoma. However, there were equally as many people with a history of melanoma who were successfully treated with Sinemet in whom there was no recurrence of melanoma. A cause-and-effect relationship between Sinemet and the recurrence of a melanoma was claimed by some and denied by others. Despite the fact that Sinemet has never been observed to stimulate melanoma, more case reports followed and the anecdotal evidence that Sinemet accelerated the growth of melanoma increased. These reports resulted in the following warning in the *Physicians' Desk Reference* (a guide that doctors use in determining which drugs might be used for treating a condition) for Sinemet:

> Because levodopa may activate a malignant melanoma, it should not be used in patients with suspicious, undiagnosed skin lesions or a history of melanoma.

This warning first appeared in 1976 and continues to be reviewed.

In 1993, Dr. William Wiener undertook a review of the reported cases of possible association between Sinemet and melanoma. In addition he reported 9 people with PD who were treated with Sinemet despite a diagnosis of melanoma. Dr. Weiner made the following points:

> If a person develops a recurrence of melanoma, the possibility must be raised that the melanoma is not a recurrence of the original melanoma but is a new primary melanoma (a melanoma unrelated to the original melanoma). It may be important, in terms of mechanisms, to distinguish, if possible, between a new melanoma that has not spread and a melanoma related to the first melanoma but one that has spread.
>
> Multiple primary melanomas (two or more melanomas with each melanoma arising on its own without a relationship to the other melanoma) may occur in up to 4% of patients with melanoma, the second melanoma usually appearing within 5 years of the original melanoma. This risk of a secondary melanoma, unrelated to the first melanoma, makes it hard to assess the role, if any, of Sinemet in aggravating melanoma.
>
> The natural history of melanoma is for late recurrence and irregular growth. It's estimated the incidence of melanoma (the number of new melanomas per year) is 9 new people with melanoma per 100,000 people. Given there are 1,000,000 people with PD, one would expect 90 new cases per year of melanoma in-patients with PD.

Dr. Wiener did not believe there is a relationship between levodopa, Sinemet, and melanoma. Two other doctors, Dr. Sober and Dr. Wick, prospectively examined 1,099 people in a study of people with melanoma and found only one person taking Sinemet. They concluded that the risk of developing melanoma could not be substantial and that there was little evidence to support a cause-and-effect relationship between melanoma and Sinemet.

At present, the evidence for a link between Sinemet and recurrence of melanoma is anecdotal and not well documented. Review of the previously reported cases that suggested such a link reveals other explanations. Several people with PD and melanoma have been successfully treated with Sinemet without a recurrence of their melanoma. With the current availability of dopamine agonists such as Mirapex and Requip—drugs not available when the initial link between Sinemet and melanoma was proposed—there are now alternatives to Sinemet in PD patients with melanoma. If the person then needs Sinemet, Sinemet should be started.

32. What else about drugs?

Compliance—the willingness to take the drugs—is an issue for many patients. Some people are in denial and do not want to admit they have PD. Taking a drug for PD is an admission of PD. This can be overcome through counseling. Remembering to take multiple doses of multiple drugs at regular and different times of the day can be a problem. This can lead to missed doses. Keeping a written schedule in your wallet or purse can help you remember which drugs you need to take and when. A pillbox with many compartments for each day is good, and a pillbox with an alarm may help even more.

The willingness to take drugs is an issue for many patients.

Cost is another issue, especially when PD is not the only disease being treated, and if you are retired and living on a fixed income, as a multidrug regimen can be expensive. Insurance may or may not cover part of the cost; thus, finding the least expensive, most effective regimen, as well as the simplest, can help with both cost and compliance. Sometimes it's a matter of just saying, "I *need* the drug;" this will help you to realize that the cost of the drug should take precedence over something else: eating out, going to the theater, or tickets to a ball game. As an example, a drug such as Comtan increases the duration of time you are "on" by at least 1.5 yours each day. In a year, if you are on Comtan, you will be "on" 547 more hours, or 23 more days. Is 23 days of being "on," of having more vitality, more zest, worth the cost?

PART FOUR

Social and Psychological Implications of PD

I have PD. Why me?

Who do I tell?

More...

33. I have PD. Why me?

No one has an answer to this question. It certainly is not anything that you did or didn't do, or anything that you had any control over; thus, you cannot blame yourself. You may wonder why you didn't see it coming, or how and why those early symptoms were never recognized for what they really were. Nothing can turn back the clock or change reality; thus, if you continue to blame yourself, ask your doctor to check to see whether you are depressed. For some people, just having a diagnosis is sufficient. Then they can sit down and discuss the prognosis and start learning as much as they can about PD. Others, especially those who have a relative with PD, may assume the worst and imagine that they will soon be disabled. Some people may be a bit too optimistic, confident that their doctor can make PD disappear with a few prescriptions. After all, we live in a time of great scientific advances, when the contributions of technology to our lives have never been greater. Thus, they reason, how is it possible that PD won't soon be cured? Obviously, a balance between unremitting pessimism and unbridled optimism must be struck. Such people, with a realistic approach, do well.

You cannot blame yourself.

34. Who do I tell?

There are no right or wrong answers. Sometimes people tell everyone they know, but others tell only the people who are closest to them. PD affects not only the person who has it, but everyone who is close to that person. Trying to hide PD may make the situation worse, adding to the anxiety, especially as the symptoms worsen and are no longer easily concealed. Telling your family and friends can be difficult, but not telling them can also cause anxiety. Who and when to

Trying to hide PD may make the situation worse.

tell are decisions that you will need to make, but hearing the news from you is better than having your family and friends guess about what is wrong with you.

PD affects both partners in a relationship. It is important to share the diagnosis with your partner as soon as possible. Facing your partner's reactions may be one of the most difficult challenges of PD. If the relationship is already shaky, the diagnosis of PD may be all that is needed to bring it to an end. But even if the relationship is on a firm foundation, a partner may still have negative reactions, denying the illness or feeling anger about how it will change the relationship. Some partners may become overprotective and smother the person with PD with too much care. Even if you have a great relationship, PD will strain it. Talk to each other—often, and about everything. Good communication is what makes the difference and will make a good relationship an even better one.

35. What do I tell my grandchildren?

Sooner or later your children or grandchildren will need to be told. How you tell them will affect how they deal with both you and PD. Keep the conversation light. Don't let your anxiety show. Let them know that it is a "natural" event, and reassure them that it isn't fatal or something contagious that they can "catch." Use language that is appropriate for their age and level of understanding. Encourage them to ask questions and share their concerns. The more accepting that you are of your condition, the more accepting the children will be, too.

In Michael J. Fox's memoir, *Lucky Man* (Hyperion: April 2002), the actor recounts explaining to his five-year-old son about his PD: "Clearly, to Sam, I was still

'Dad,' just 'Dad with the wiggly hand.' Was it possible that I could look at things the same way, that I was still me—just me plus Parkinson?"

When you are ready to inform your children or grand-children of your PD, you may be surprised—as Fox was—at the inspiration that can be drawn from this difficult moment.

36. Do I tell my boss?

This depends on several factors and especially on what kind of job you have and your relationship with your boss. Will PD affect your job performance? An airline pilot or a surgeon will have to tell his or her employer sooner than someone who works in sales. How your boss responds may not be predictable either. Although PD is a disability and federal law prohibits firing a person because of a disability, you could be reassigned to a different job or be pressured into taking early retirement. Then again, an employer might be willing to make accommodations to keep you or even allow you to work from home. For many people, their job helps them to feel defined—what they do is who they are. Finding yourself without your occupational defini-tion of self—regardless of how gently you are let go or with what allowances—can be a terrible blow. Finding another way to use your skills and knowledge will lead to new ways of being productive and can restore your sense of identity. Other people may be close enough to retirement when they are diagnosed with PD that they are grateful for the excuse to retire and do things that they have waited for years to do.

37. Will I be able to drive?

Driving is the one common ritual that measures maturity and independence. As a teen, getting a driver's license is a major milestone of independence. Giving up driving is, for some people, equivalent to losing their freedom and independence. Can a person with PD continue to drive? Early in PD driving should pose no problem as long as symptoms are mild and don't interfere with your ability to react to traffic situations. As symptoms progress, however, decreased motor skills and concentration may compromise your ability to drive. When muscle rigidity and lack of coordination make it difficult to react quickly, the reality of the situation must be faced, and the decision to drive must be reconsidered. If there is any question about driving skills and abilities, a professional driving instructor can evaluate the situation.

A loss of driving does not necessarily mean a loss of independence or isolation: Not driving doesn't mean not going places. Take stock of all of the available options: a partner who is happy to drive, a friend who is willing to accompany you to appointments, and public transportation. If you no longer have the expense of maintaining a car and insurance, the price of a taxi ride is a bargain. It may take a bit more planning to arrange, but don't give up on going places because you can't drive.

38. What about my social life?

Staying connected with other people is vital. It is easy to feel embarrassed about the symptoms of PD and withdraw. This only leads to isolation and depression.

When you give in to PD, you become its victim, suffering embarrassment and loneliness. When you accept that PD is a reality in your life, you can find ways of coping, thus regaining a sense of control and getting on with living your life. Remaining active with social events, going to church, going to the theater or concerts, and entertaining at home may take a bit more effort, but are worth it. It is important to interact with others and to share your thoughts and your hopes and dreams. Join a gym and exercise regularly—it will help you to stay in shape as well as get you out with other people. Take up yoga; it will calm your mind as it stretches and keeps your muscles limber. Members of a support group offer camaraderie and will share their own methods of coping. It is also important to be on top of the newest information: try *www.Parkinson.org.*

39. What about sex?

Just how PD contributes to loss of desire and its impact on sexuality is still not clear. It's not uncommon for sexual desires to decrease in later life—but because PD does affect the autonomic nervous system, it may lessen the response to sexual stimulation. For women, menopause brings hormonal changes, and some women experience a decreased desire for sexual relationships. However, a woman with PD may also feel that her symptoms have robbed her of her femininity and may feel less attractive and less desirable as a sexual partner. For older men, sexual dysfunction or the inability to achieve or maintain an erection can affect their sense of self-esteem. Men who believe that their sexual prowess is the emblem of their manhood feel that this loss is the ultimate humiliation. Still, many men and women remain sexually interested and active all their lives.

PD does not mean giving up sex. You and your partner have many options for improving your sex lives. First, start talking with your partner about your needs and feelings. If your partner is your caregiver, he or she may be so caught up in day-to-day concerns that sex is the last thing on his or her mind. If you have had a close relationship, try to restore a bit of romance into your lives. Be sure to adhere to your medication schedule, exercise regularly, eat balanced meals, and keep yourself in the best possible shape, as this will reduce symptoms and their impact on your sexuality. Put satin sheets on the bed, as they will make turning over in bed easier. If your "off" times interfere, perhaps you can "plan" your encounters for times when you know that your medications will be working and you will be "on." Yes, it does reduce the spontaneity, but thinking about it while waiting may actually build the anticipation and increase the pleasure. If sexual dysfunction or incontinence is a problem, talk with your doctor. If despite everything you and your partner cannot satisfy each other, a skilled mental health or sex therapist can often work with couples to resolve their difficulties.

40. What else can I do to cope with PD?

PD does impose major lifestyle changes, and it is easy to feel an overwhelming sense of loss. You can no longer do many things as easily as you did before, or perhaps you may not be able to do them at all. Although PD may define what you can and cannot do, it does not define you. You are *not* your disease. You can regain a measure of control by making a list of all of the things that you can do. Then make another list of all the things that you can do to care of yourself, such as diet, exercise, managing stress, and taking your drugs on time. Perhaps one of the most difficult hurdles is learning to accept help from others. Because PD will make you unable to do certain things, you will need help. Learn to accept help gracefully, without losing your dignity. Giving help has its own rewards, one of which is an offer of appreciation.

Another difficulty is responding to the unkind looks or remarks from others, particularly strangers. Although they may never have known anyone with PD, their rudeness or pity is unwelcome. Education—improving public awareness and media coverage or making information about PD available to others—is important. If you have the opportunity and the courage, you could explain to them that you have a neurologic disorder that affects your walking and balance. The Parkinson Disease Society of Great Britain has a small card that can be handed to people that says: *I have Parkinson disease. I may be slow to move or unsteady on my feet. I may have difficulty speaking and writing clearly. I can hear and understand you. Please allow time.*

Staying active and interacting with others give opportunities for expanding your horizons and staying in touch with others. Find, join, and attend PD support groups, which offer camaraderie with other folks who have gone down the same path as you, who know how PD feels, and who can share with you their best methods of coping. They are also an excellent source of knowledge about PD and can keep you posted on the best books and web pages or the newest developments in research and treatment of PD. Friends made in support groups can keep you from feeling alone in your circumstances.

As symptoms progress, it will be necessary to revise your expectations of yourself. Insisting on doing things or driving yourself to places the way that you used to will bring on increased stress and anxiety. Your successes and accomplishments prior to having PD are not realistic goals now. Adjust your priorities accordingly. Set goals for yourself that are attainable and challenging but that can be accomplished within your physical and emotional limits. Remember past successes, as those memories can be inspiring when you don't feel encouraged. Focus on small victories, and keep track of them. Reward yourself as you meet each goal. Progress will also keep your spirits up and keep you feeling in control of your life. Your accomplishments will bolster your self-esteem.

41. As a caregiver, how can I cope with my partner's PD?

As a partner of someone with PD, you never expected to be in this situation, and you may feel unprepared for your new responsibilities. Frustration, anger, resentment, fear, sadness, and hopelessness may all rush over you, and then you may feel guilty for having these emotions! Life seems to be spinning out of control. Like your PD partner, you need to accept this situation because PD is something over which you have no control. When you accept this, you can focus on parts of your life over which you do have control, where you can establish some kind of order and impose some kind of schedule to regain a saner perspective. The balance of your relationship is shifting; you will be challenged emotionally, spiritually, and physically. A partner who mowed the lawn and kept the garden may no longer be able to perform these tasks. A partner who shopped and cooked and cleaned the house may have to share those tasks with his or her mate. At times, the responsibility for the home combined with caregiving for the ill partner can become so burdensome that you feel pushed beyond your abilities to cope.

As a caregiver you must take care of yourself physically by eating a balanced diet and getting enough sleep and regular exercise. Exercise is a great way to relieve stress while strengthening you for the physical challenges of caregiving. Take care of yourself emotionally by learning to channel your emotions and feelings into constructive outlets. Find a support group for caregivers. Talk about your feelings with friends and family. Learn as much about PD as possible so that the next challenge won't come as such a surprise. Take time to do the things that you enjoy: Go for a walk or spend time with nature or meet a friend for lunch. Don't neglect your spiritual side either; connect with your higher power and meditate or pray every day. Let your spirituality give you strength.

When your workload feels impossible, it probably is. Rally your resources, gather family and friends to give you a hand, or check on resources that are available in your community. Hire some help so that your time is spent where it is needed most. Maybe you need to adjust your expectations a bit—you may be setting too high a standard for yourself. Perfection is not necessary, and a burned-out caregiver is not able to care for anyone.

To be a good caregiver sometimes means allowing the person with PD to be independent. It may be easier and faster for *you* to do something, but remember that your partner may still be able to do many things—it just takes longer. Encourage him or her to be independent and active and to do as much as possible independently. There may be times when the best you can do is merely to be there, to sit beside your partner, to hold hands, or to lend your moral support and give the warmth of your presence.

PART FIVE

Progression

What stage am I in?

How do I know if I'm worse?

My dose of Sinemet no longer works.
What's happening?

More . . .

42. What stage am I in?

Because not all people have the same symptoms at the same time, measuring their progression can be difficult. A number of rating scales are presently available. The simplest and most widely used is the Hoehn and Yahr staging scale (Table 1). It divides PD into five categories, from early, one-sided effects to full disability. In the early research for which this scale was designed, the goal was to measure the years between the development of each stage. The findings showed that the progression was not uniform; some people progressed rapidly and some slowly.

The second measurement tool (the most commonly used) is the Unified Parkinson Disease Rating Scale. It uses a four-point scoring system and measures a standardized core of 42 assessments in four broad categories: mental states such as mood and behavior, activities of daily living, motor responses, and the complications of treatment.

Table 1   Modified Hoen and Yahr staging

Stage 0	No signs of disease
Stage 1	Unilateral disease
Stage 2	Bilateral disease, no difficulty walking
Stage 3	Bilateral disease, minimal difficulty walking
Stage 4	Bilateral disease, moderate difficulty walking
Stage 5	Bilateral disease, unable to walk

43. How do I know if I'm worse?

If you were initially put on Sinemet, one of the first things that you'll notice is that your doses of Sinemet no longer "kick in" or last as long. You become aware that your last dose of Sinemet has worn off before your next dose, leaving you slow, stiff, or aching. At this point in your disease, doses of Sinemet gradually wear off, or sometimes they abruptly stop working as though a switch inside of you was turned off. If you were taking three Sinemet doses a day, you may now need four or more doses. If you could miss one or more doses without symptoms, you now can't miss any dose. If initially you were started on a dopamine agonist (Mirapex, Requip, or Permax) and did well, you may now need Sinemet in addition to the agonist.

44. My dose of Sinemet no longer works. What's happening?

Sinemet has a short half-life (a measure of its duration of action) and is delivered in pulses, irregularly and discontinuously, to the brain. This pulsatile and irregular delivery of Sinemet is partly responsible for wearing off or "turning off" (usually called on-off). This is also discussed in Question 27. The irregular delivery of Sinemet may be partly improved by adding Comtan. Comtan increases Sinemet's duration of action. The irregular delivery may be improved, in part, by adding a dopamine agonist. An agonist (Mirapex, Requip, Permax) provides the brain with an alternate to dopamine. Although the irregular delivery of Sinemet is partly responsible for wearing off or for on-off, it is the progression of PD with continued loss of dopamine-producing cells in the brain that is mainly responsible for wearing off and on-off. Sinemet's effectiveness depends on the ability of the remaining dopamine cells to change L-dopa to dopamine, an ability that is compromised as each remaining cell disappears. The effectiveness of the agonists does not depend on the ability of the remaining cells to change L-dopa to dopamine. That is why, in addition to their being used as the first treatment for PD, they're also used in more advanced PD. Finding the proper balance between Sinemet, Sinemet plus Comtan, and an agonist requires time and patience. Keeping a daily diary detailing when you take your medication, when you eat, and whether you are on (medication working) or off (medication not working) will give you and your doctor a powerful insight into what is happening.

Sometimes if you miss a dose of Sinemet, especially at night, you may experience a painful cramping in the muscles of one or both of your legs. The cramping (called dystonia) is usually worse in the early morning before your first dose of medication. Adding a dopamine agonist at night or taking a dose of Sinemet before getting out of bed usually helps. It's not that your Sinemet no longer works—it will always work to some extent— it's that it no longer works as well as in the beginning. Hey! Nothing, from cars to human beings, works as well when it's older as when it was younger. PD is a biological phenomenon, it gets worse with time, but there are certainly ways of overcoming this.

45. I can't move. What's happening?

The sudden and seemingly unpredictable "off" time is called freezing. Freezing is also discussed in Question 27. Freezing may have a pattern, and you may be able to control it by adjusting your medication. If you keep a

24-hour diary, this may give you and your doctor a clue as to why you're freezing and how to adjust your drugs.

Sometimes freezing doesn't respond to drugs. In these cases, the freezing occurs, in part, because a center in your brain (one that automatically adjusts the length and rhythm of your stride) isn't working. As you change, or think about changing, the length and rhythm of your stride while turning or walking into a room or approaching a curb, your feet shut down, and you freeze. Freezing, if it was not present before, indicates progression of PD. But as with most symptoms of progression, there are ways around freezing. Don't panic! Anxiety, fear, or panic makes things worse: the more that you try to move and can't, the more anxious you get, the more frustrated you will become and the more your feet will stick to the ground. Restoring the rhythm of your stride by stepping over a real or imaginary line helps.

46. I move too much. What's happening?

The twisting, turning, dance-like movements are called dyskinesia. This is also discussed in Question 27. This is what's happening to Michael J. Fox. Two types of dyskinesia exist: dyskinesias that appear as Sinemet reaches its peak effect (called peak-dose dyskinesia) and dyskinesias that appear at the start or at the end of a dose of Sinemet (before the next dose is due, called diphasic dyskinesias). Most people learn to live with their peak-dose dyskinesia if the dyskinesias don't interfere with their daily activities. Decreasing your dose of Sinemet may decrease your dyskinesia, but at a price: You may not be able to move. Treatment consists of gradually replacing part of your daily dose of Sinemet with a dopamine agonist (Mirapex, Requip, or Permax). Stopping deprenyl (selegiline), a drug that prolongs Sinemet's duration of action, may help. Deprenyl is long acting, and its effect on Sinemet is variable and sometimes unpredictable. Stopping it results in a more predictable, although shorter, duration of action of Sinemet. This, in turn, makes it easier to regulate dyskinesias. Comtan, a drug that also prolongs Sinemet's duration of action, is short acting, and its effect on Sinemet is predictable. If you're taking Comtan with each dose of Sinemet and you're having peak-dose dyskinesia, eliminating one or more doses of Comtan may help. Adding amantadine (Symmetrel) may decrease peak-dose dyskinesia. The reason is unclear. Peak-dose dyskinesias severe enough to interfere with daily activities and unresponsive to the previously mentioned treatments usually respond to deep brain stimulation (see Question 70).

Diphasic dyskinesias are usually more severe, more difficult to treat, and more difficult to recognize. Thus, from watching Michael J. Fox on television, it is impossible to say whether he has peak-dose or diphasic dyskinesia, or both. Keeping a 24-hour diary helps distinguish diphasic from peak-dose dyskinesia. If the diphasic dyskinesias are mild, adding a dopamine agonist, increasing the frequency with which you take Sinemet, or adding Comtan by sustaining the length of time that you're on may decrease the dyskinesias. However, increasing the frequency with which you take Sinemet or adding Comtan may increase peak-dose dyskinesias. Because the treatment for diphasic dyskinesias is different from peak-dose dyskinesia and because people usually have both, treatment is difficult and not always satisfactory.

Dyskinesia results from treatment with Sinemet and from progression of the underlying disease. Sinemet has a short duration of action and is delivered in pulses—irregularly and discontinuously—to the brain. This irregular delivery of Sinemet is responsible, in part, for wearing off or on-off and dyskinesia. Sinemet sensitizes the dopamine receptors on cells in a region called the striatum. There are five types of dopamine receptors, and two types (called D–1 and D–2) are in the striatum. The dopamine agonists (Mirapex, Requip, Permax) stimulate the D–2 receptors. Dopamine (made from Sinemet) stimulates the D–1 and D–2 receptors. Pulsatile, irregular stimulation of the D–1 receptors is responsible in part for peak-dose and diphasic dyskinesia. As PD progresses, such stimulation results in overactivity of cells in two other regions: the **globus pallidus** and the **subthalamic nucleus**.

Prevention is the best treatment for dyskinesias. This fact has led doctors to start newly diagnosed people on dopamine agonists: agonists such as Mirapex and Requip are long-acting, are delivered more continuously, do not stimulate the D–1 receptors, and when used alone, rarely cause dyskinesias. If peak-dose or diphasic dyskinesia interferes with daily activities, deep brain stimulation is an option (see Question 70). Dyskinesia results from overactivity of the globus pallidus and subthalamic nucleus. DBS decreases this overactivity. Dyskinesia does not necessarily mean PD is progressing. Dyskinesia is more a symptom of dopamine sensitivity than of PD progression.

47. Why do I fall?

Falls occur in people with PD and can result in injuries: fractured ankles, hips, shoulders and skulls. Falls result from postural instability, or loss of "righting

Globus pallidus
a region of the basal ganglia affected in PD. This region of the brain is known to be overactive in animal models of PD.

Subthalamic nucleus
a region of the brain located below the thalamus that acts as "brake" on the substantia nigra.

reflexes," an inability to "right oneself," or to take corrective measures to prevent a fall. Falls usually occur late in PD (5 to 10 years after PD is diagnosed). Falls early in PD usually indicate a PD-like disorder, but not PD. In PD, falls may occur as a result of drugs. Thus, as a dose of Sinemet wears off, your steps become shorter and shorter (called festination), and you may trip over your own feet. Such falls may be accompanied by freezing, in which your legs lock up. Such falls may be helped by adjusting your drugs—for example, adding Comtan or a dopamine agonist such as Mirapex or Requip. In PD, falls may occur as a result of overmedication: dyskinesia. Here, you lose control of your legs, your legs fly out from you. Adjusting your drugs may be beneficial. If this does not help, then surgery, DBS, may be an option.

In many people with PD, falls occur independently of drugs, unrelated to freezing. As PD progresses, postural instability—loss of your righting reflexes—appears as a separate condition. For example, suppose you're standing and someone pushes or shoves you backward. Your feet lunge backward, but your body and head, without you thinking about it, lunge forward, correcting for the "lunge" backward, preventing you from falling. The correction takes place because your righting reflexes are working. They sensed the sudden displacement of your feet, the "lunge" backward. They sensed not only that you were moving backward but also the speed with which you were moving and relayed this information to centers in your brain, centers that reacted quicker than you can think. These centers then "commanded" your body and head to lunge forward, correcting for the lunge backward. Sometimes there's a delay, and you take, without thinking about it, one or two steps backward before correcting yourself. If you have PD, your righting reflexes may slow down, and you cannot take corrective action quickly. Thus, in response to being pushed or shoved backward, you topple backward like a tree.

Your ability to take such corrective action depends on information from your eyes, sensors in your feet (called "position sense"), and sensors in your inner ears ("motion sense"). Each of these sensors—your eyes, your position sense, your inner ears—are working; however, the center (or centers) for the righting reflex, which integrates and reacts to this information, is defective in PD.

Your vision plays a role in balance. Its role is to compensate for defects in position sense and motion sense. If your position sense is defective or if your feet cannot sense where they are, such as occur in the neuropathy of diabetes or in vitamin B12 deficiency, your eyes can compensate for your feet. A diabetic with **neuropathy** (damage to the nerves in feet) or a person who is deficient in vitamin B12 can stand without swaying or falling if his or her eyes are open; however, if he or she closes his or her eyes or stands or walks in the dark, his or her feet are no longer directed by his eyes, thus causing a fall. The person topples like a tree because his or her righting reflexes no longer receive the information that they need to maintain his balance. A blind person who has normal position sense and normal motion sense is able to stand and walk with perfect balance and does not fall unless he or she trips or bumps into something. If the person trips because his or her righting reflexes are working, corrective measures can be taken to break the fall; thus, the person does not topple like someone with PD.

Neuropathy
damage to the nerves in the hands and feet.

Your inner ears play a role in balance. The inner ears monitor "motion sense" and allow you to maintain your balance when you suddenly change position, as in turning. In turning, motion sensors are activated in your inner ears, and messages go from them to a region of the brainstem called the **vestibular nucleus**. From here, the messages go to a region called the cerebellum, which acts as a coordinating center. The vestibular nuclei and the cerebellum respond to changes in movement. They relay such information to higher centers in your brain, which in turn relay the information directly to your legs. Think of an attack on an army unit in a foreign country. News of the attack (the equivalent of a change in motion) is relayed to a local command post (the equivalent of the vestibular nuclei and cerebellum) and headquarters in Washington (the higher centers in the brain). Knowing that there will be a delay while Washington "digests" the information, the local command post (the vestibular nuclei and cerebellum) will direct the first response.

Postural instability in PD is tested by having you stand with your arms at your side, your feet comfortably apart, and your eyes open. The doctor stands behind you and suddenly pulls you backward. Your response to such a displacement is rated as follows: 0 = normal, no displacement; 1 = recovers unaided; 2 = would fall if not caught; 3 = falls spontaneously; and 4 = unable to stand without support.

Your feet play a role in balance. Position sense sensors in your feet attached to nerves that run up your legs monitor your position in space. Position sense is tested by asking you to stand, arms at your side, feet comfortably apart, eyes wide open, and noting whether you

Vestibular nucleus

a region of the brain stem that receives messages from the inner ears regarding balance.

sway forward or backward or side to side. The test is then repeated with your eyes closed. This is called the **Romberg test**, after the neurologist who first described it. The information from your feet is relayed up your legs to your spinal cord. Here the information is carried to a region called the **thalamus**. The thalamus is on level with the **basal ganglia** (a series of inter-connected regions of the brain including the striatum, globus pallidus, and thalamus). Your left thalamus monitors information from the right side of your body, and your right thalamus monitors information from the left side of your body. This information is not consciously appreciated. Fibers from your right thalamus go to the right side of your cortex (where it is consciously appreciated). Fibers from your left thalamus go to the left side of your cortex (where it is consciously appreciated).

In order to make the necessary corrective movements in response to turning, or being pulled or pushed, the corrective movements must be made quickly before you're consciously aware of being pulled or pushed. These movements may be initiated in the thalamus. The thalamus already receives messages from the vestibular nuclei and the cerebellum. The basal ganglia, which includes the substantia nigra, the subthalamic nucleus, the striatum, and the globus pallidus, all of the structures involved in PD, also send messages to the thalamus. The thalamus is thus uniquely positioned to be the center for righting reflexes. It's thought that the person with PD and postural instability has a vestibular deficit, a cerebellar deficit, and a position sense deficit, deficits of which he or she is not aware. These deficits are at the level of the thalamus: above the vestibular nuclei, above the cerebellum, and

Progression

Romberg test

a test that observes whether a person asked to stand still sways backward or forward with eyes open, then with eyes closed.

Thalamus

region of the brain that receives impulses from the senses and transmits them to the conscious brain.

Basal ganglia

a series of inter-connected regions of the brain including the striatum, globus pallidus, and thalamus.

above the posterior nuclei and columns. At this time, we are unable to treat this deficit with drugs. Treatment is education: teaching you the limits of what you can do and teaching you how to compensate.

48. Is the pain I have experienced part of PD?

It is said that pain and PD don't go together; thus, pain appears to be something else, such as arthritis, bursitis, a bad back, or a frozen shoulder. However, pain is part of PD and has many forms. How common is pain is PD? Perhaps 50% of people with PD complain of pain at one time, and in perhaps 50% of them—25% of all people with PD—the pain is related to PD and not to something else. The pain may be related to PD if it fits a pattern, if it's worse where PD is worse, if it's relieved by PD drugs, or if there's no other cause.

In the beginning, before you're diagnosed with PD, you may complain of a dull pain, like a sprain. The pain may be described as aching, gnawing, or nagging. The pain is usually confined to a shoulder, the neck, the back, or a hip. These are either major weight-bearing regions (the back and the hip) or the shoulders. This pain is probably related to the rigidity of PD, which results in the muscles becoming stiffer, less elastic, and harder and more painful to move. This type of pain magically disappears when Sinemet or a dopamine agonist is started. Later, you may complain of a cramping, sharp, stabbing, or throbbing pain. The pain is usually confined to one or both calves, forearms, thighs, or upper arms. This pain is probably related to the dystonia of PD, which results in the muscles becoming hard. This pain magically disappears when a dopamine agonist is started. Dystonia is different from rigidity. Although both make the muscles hard, in rigidity, the hardness results from the muscles becoming less elastic, whereas in dystonia, it results from the muscles contracting without relaxing. Dystonia of the calves, forearms, thigh, or upper arms may be an early symptom of PD, usually in people who are less than 40 years old. It may appear in people with PD who are taking Sinemet. Usually it appears as Sinemet wears off, typically in the early morning when Sinemet levels are low. This is called an "off dystonia." It's worse on the side that is more affected by PD. It's treated by adding a dopamine agonist. The pain of dystonia can appear as Sinemet peaks, called "on dystonia." It's harder to treat, thus requiring you to rearrange all of your drugs to reduce the highs and lows of Sinemet.

If you feel pain, only you can describe it. Be as specific as you can. Asking the following questions is helpful:

- *Location.* Where does it hurt most? The shoulder? The hip? The back? Does it stay in one place, or does it radiate? If so, where?
- *Intensity.* How bad is it? Describe it on a scale of 0 to 10, where 0 is no pain and 10 feels as if your arm (or leg) was yanked off or your skin was ripped off. The pain of PD is usually a 4 to 7. It's never a 10.
- *Duration.* How long have you had the pain? Hours? Days? Weeks? Years? During a typical day, how long does it last?
- *Associations.* Is the pain associated with inflammation, redness, swelling, or warmth of the overlying skin? The pain of PD shouldn't be associated with any of these.
- *Position.* What positions, if any, make it better? What, if any, make it worse?

- *Quality.* Words used to describe the pain include aching, biting, burning, cramping (like a Charlie-horse), gripping (like being caught in between a pair of pliers), hurting, nipping, pinching, ripping, smarting, stabbing, and throbbing. A diffuse, not well-localized burning or throbbing pain may sometimes occur in an arm or a leg or across the chest. Whether this is related to PD, anxiety, or depression is difficult to pin down. It probably results from a disorder of the autonomic nervous system.

49. I can't sleep. Is this PD or am I anxious or depressed?

Anxiety and depression are common in PD and can interfere with sleep; however, insomnia (difficulty falling asleep or difficulty staying asleep or both) is part of PD.

It is normal during sleep for people to awaken during the night—to roll over, to change positions, and then to fall back to sleep without any problem. People with PD may awaken and find themselves so stiff that they are unable to make such adjustments and then can't go back to sleep. The problem may be that your last dose of Sinemet wasn't enough to give you the mobility that you need in bed to sleep through the night. This problem can be helped by adding Comtan or a dopamine agonist. Insomnia consists of one or more of the following: difficulty falling asleep, difficulty remaining asleep, frequent nighttime awakenings, early-morning awakening, and unrefreshing sleep.

Temporary insomnia lasting less than 4 weeks is self-limited and has no serious repercussions. It occurs in up to 50% of all people and is more frequent in older people, shift workers, international travelers, and people who are under stress. Chronic insomnia, such as occurs in PD, lasts longer than 4 weeks, is not self-limited, and may have repercussions. Such insomnia usually results in daytime fatigue, grogginess, irritability, mood swings, and difficulty paying attention or concentrating. People with chronic insomnia are more likely to suffer from anxiety, depression, mood swings, or paranoia. Whether these disorders came first and insomnia is part of them or whether the insomnia came first and unmasked them is a source of debate. In discussing insomnia with your doctor, you should be prepared to answer questions such as these:

- What time do you go to bed? Before midnight? After midnight?
- How long does it take for you to fall asleep? Less than an hour? More than an hour?
- While trying to fall asleep, what do you do? Read? Listen to the radio? Watch TV? Worry? Stare into space?
- Do you wake up during the night? For what reason? Bad dream? Going to the bathroom? Worry? Restless legs? No reason?
- How many times do you wake up? Once? More than once?
- How many hours do you sleep? Four hours? Two hours?
- When do usually wake up? Before 4:00 a.m.? After 4:00 a.m.?
- After you wake up, do you get out of or stay in bed? How long? Less than an hour? More than an hour?
- When you wake up, are you refreshed? Or groggy?
- Do you nap during the day? Once? More than once?

If you have a bed partner, he or she can be a valuable source of information because most people are unaware of their behavior while sleeping. Your bed partner is probably the only one who can comment on specific behaviors: talking in your sleep, crying out or shouting during sleep, snoring (which may indicate sleep apnea), thrashing or kicking while asleep, or walking in your sleep.

Such preparation will help you and your doctor to identify the cause (or causes) of your insomnia. Just telling your doctor that you can't sleep without first analyzing your sleep habits is not helpful.

Temporary insomnia may be caused by anxiety (worry over family, friends, business), situational adjustments (new bed, strange bed, new house, new job, new bed partner), sleep–wake disruptions (change in schedule, international jet travel), or a new drug. Once the cause of insomnia is identified, corrective measures can be taken, and the insomnia will disappear.

Chronic insomnia has many causes, which may include the following:

- Heart and lung disease.
- Kidney, prostate, and bladder disease.
- Endocrine disorders such as an overactive thyroid gland or diabetes.
- Sleep apnea (this results from decreased tone of the muscles of the roof of your mouth, which in turn, results in your uvula falling back into your throat and partially blocking your airway when you lay down).
- PD drugs such as deprenyl and amantadine.
- Drugs for other conditions such as sleeping pills, which may, paradoxically, worsen insomnia if used improperly or withdrawn inappropriately.

Many people with PD have insomnia. This may be related to a primary sleep disorder that arises from an as yet unknown disturbance in sleep rhythm. The centers regulating sleep are in the brainstem, a region uniquely positioned to regulate sleep as it regulates eye opening and closing, posture, and tone. The centers regulating sleep are located near the substantia nigra, the region most affected in PD. Thus, it's not surprising that there is an association between PD and difficulty sleeping. The diagnosis of a primary sleep disorder is made in the absence of other causes of insomnia. Sometimes the diagnosis of a primary sleep disorder requires evaluation in a sleep laboratory. If such a disorder causes insomnia, initial treatment is to provide you with information about sleep and to instruct you in such simple and effective measures as to go to bed only when you're sleepy; to leave your bedroom if you're unable to fall asleep within 30 minutes or if you wake up and can't get back to sleep within 30 minutes and to return only when you're sleepy; to wake up at the same time every morning, including weekends; and to avoid daytime naps.

Relaxation techniques are helpful. Examples include neck muscle relaxation and diaphragmatic breathing. Some people with insomnia without realizing it engage in activities that aggravate the problem: excessive use of stimulants such as coffee or caffeine-containing soft drinks, sleeping excessively on weekends, or daytime napping.

Many people with insomnia become anxious and preoccupied with their difficulty sleeping, and because worry and concern tend to peak around bedtime, this worsens the insomnia. If education and instructions in proper sleep hygiene are insufficient, the next approach is short-term use of a prescription or nonprescription drug. Your doctor must decide on the proper drugs or combination of drugs. Commonly used nonprescription, over-the-counter drugs include the following: kava root, usually up to 500 mg per night; melatonin, a hormone secreted by the pineal gland and thought to regulate circadian rhythms, usually 1 to 3 mg per night; and valerian root, usually 500 mg per night. These drugs, although not requiring a prescription, may like other drugs have side effects and interact with prescription drugs. *You must tell your doctor about **all** of the drugs that you are taking.*

Commonly used prescription drugs include benzodiazepines, a class of drugs that bind to a special receptor in the brain, called the benzodiazepine receptor; nonbenzodiazepine sleep medications, a class of drugs that are not benzodiazepines but that bind to the benzodiazepine receptors; and antidepressants with sleep-inducing properties. Some drugs have a long half-life, reflecting delayed metabolism by the body. Such drugs are likely to cause daytime grogginess or drowsiness. Examples include Elavil, Norpramin, and Sinequan.

50. My partner kicks and screams in his sleep. Is he crazy?

No! But he may have a disorder of rapid eye movement (REM) sleep. Vivid and frightening dreams dominate; thus, your partner may kick and scream as if running away from something, but after waking, he remembers nothing. REM sleep disorders are more disturbing to you than to your partner. Typically, dreaming occurs during a phase of sleep called REM (when the eyes are moving). Muscle tone during REM sleep is minimal, which stops your partner from acting out his dreams. During disordered REM sleep, your partner's dreams are vivid, often violent, and his muscle tone is increased, allowing dreams to be acted out, resulting in screaming, kicking, or punching, as though he is fighting someone. Disorders in REM sleep can result from the effects of Sinemet or dopamine agonists on the brain. They can be treated by reducing the amount of PD drugs or adding a drug such as Seroquel, or Geodon, or Clozaril, drugs that dampen, in part, the actions of PD drugs.

51. My legs ache, and I'm constantly moving them. Why?

Restless legs syndrome (RLS) is an uncomfortable, aching sensation that is relieved if you constantly move your legs. RLS occurs in the evening or at night when you're resting. The sensations are described as an irresistible urge to move as twitching, burning, stabbing, creeping and crawling, aching, heaviness, and tension felt deep in the calf muscles or even the bones. Occasionally, the sensation spreads to the feet or the thighs, but rarely to the arms or hands. The only relief is to get up and walk, which for someone with PD can be difficult. Insomnia often follows, leading to more problems with a lack of sleep, anxiety, or depression.

Restless legs syndrome

an uncomfortable, aching sensation that is relieved if you constantly move your legs; usually occurs during sleep or while resting.

RLS affects approximately 5% of the U.S. population and is often unrecognized and misdiagnosed. Although it affects up to 5% of the population, in only 10% is RLS sufficiently bothersome for people to seek treatment. Although RLS may begin at any age, but most people affected are 50 and older. Approximately 80% of people with RLS may have periodic limb movements (called myoclonus) during sleep. Myoclonus occurs rhythmically and is not harmful but can be frightening—especially to your bed partner.

Diabetes, iron deficiency anemia, kidney disease, peripheral neuropathy, and poor circulation may cause RLS. Most of the time the cause is unknown. RLS is related, in part, to abnormalities in dopamine. Dopamine agonists help RLS, and dopamine antagonists worsen RLS. Although there is link with dopamine and although restless legs are common in people with PD, a debate exists about whether restless legs are part of PD.

The dopamine agonists Mirapex and Requip are effective in the treatment of PD and restless legs (secondary to PD or unrelated to PD). Mirapex is started at 0.125 mg at bedtime and is gradually increased to a maximum of 1.5 mg three times daily for PD or restless legs. Requip is started at 0.25 mg and is increased to 3 to 8 mg three times daily for PD or restless legs.

52. Why can't I read anymore?

You may have excellent vision, but reading is difficult. In PD, the muscles of your eyes slow down and may be less able to accommodate for the rapid movements that are necessary for scanning a line of print. Occasionally, you may have double vision. This condition, related to PD, may be helped by using specially designed prisms. A second condition related to PD may involve interpretation of the images cast on the retina by the lens of your eye. The retina contains dopamine cells, and when the dopamine system is affected in PD, it may influence your eyes. A third condition may be the lack of eye blinking. Your eyes may become dry and irritated because your lids do not blink enough to wash away dust, pollen, or other irritants. This condition may be helped with artificial tears.

If you have difficulty seeing, consult an ophthalmologist, a medical doctor who can diagnose and treat eye conditions. Remember that you are more likely to have difficulty seeing because of conditions unrelated to PD. The eye doctor will check your visual acuity for both distance (far) vision and near (reading) vision. A common condition is **presbyopia** where the length of your lens changes with age and in order to read you're forced to hold the paper further and further away). A second condition is **cataracts**, in which the lens of your eye becomes cloudy, and you think you're looking through "water." A third condition is **glaucoma**, which results from an accumulation of fluid behind the eye. The fluid presses on the optic nerves and can, in time, lead to blindness. Pain often accompanies acute glaucoma. Chronic glaucoma is usually silent—that is, you may not know you have it. Certain PD drugs, the anticholinergic drugs such as Artane and Cogentin, can increase eye pressure—especially in people with narrow-angle glaucoma.

The doctor will check the pressure in your eye to determine whether you have glaucoma. Then, using an ophthalmoscope, he or she will look at the back of your eye, the retina. The retina is the only place in the body where the arteries (as distinct from the veins) can be examined. Looking at the arteries of the eye provides a "window" into all of the arteries elsewhere. Such information is especially helpful if you have diabetes or high blood pressure, conditions that affect the

Presbyopia

a condition of the eye in which the length of the lens changes with age.

Cataracts

a condition in which the lens of the eye becomes cloudy and obscured, usually relieved with surgery.

Glaucoma

a disease of the eyes in which fluid accumulates behind the eye and presses on the optic nerve, in time causing blindness.

arteries. Other retinal conditions that can be diagnosed with an ophthalmoscope include macular degeneration.

53. Is depression part of PD?

Approximately 50% of people with PD suffer from depression. In some, depression is the first symptom of PD. People with PD may suffer from an endogenous depression, a depression unrelated to any external event. Such depressions are part of the chemical imbalance underlying PD, and some studies have shown that the PD drug Mirapex can also act as an anti-depressant in some people with this kind of biochemical depression, even if they don't have PD. People with PD can also suffer from an exogenous depression, a depression related to external events such as job loss, retirement, or knowledge of a relative with advanced PD with fear of becoming as disabled as the relative. In some people, depression is associated with anxiety, and in some, the anxiety is so overwhelming that agitated depression is a result. Depression is sometimes associated with a sleep disorder: an inability to fall asleep at night, prolonged sleeping during the day, or a combination of both. In some, depression is associated with a passive, quiet, and withdrawn state and can be treated in several ways and will depend on some of the associated factors described previously here.

How do you know if you're depressed? Sometimes trying to determine whether you're depressed or whether you have PD or both is difficult. Someone with PD who has a sad, poker face, a soft, weepy voice, and a stooped posture (bent as though bearing the weight of the world on his or her shoulders) may appear depressed when he or she is not. Conversely, a depressed person who moves slowly, speaks softly, and walks stooped over may appear to have PD when he or she does not. You may be depressed if during the past week you have cried for no apparent reason; have felt sad, helpless, or guilt stricken; had difficulty sleeping at night or have slept all day; have felt anxious, fearful, uncertain, or worried for no apparent reason; have lost interest in your work, hobbies, family, or friends; and have began to drink alcohol heavily.

The Depression Questionnaire (Table 2) may help you determine whether you're depressed. The questionnaire is modeled on the Hamilton Depression Scale and has not been validated as a test; rather, it is meant as a teaching guide. If during the past week you have had one of the following symptoms on 4 or more days, select "Yes"; if you have not, select "No."

If you answered yes to 10 or more questions, then you are probably depressed. If you answered yes to 15 or more questions, then you are depressed. Discuss this with your spouse, family, minister, and doctor. If you have thought of ending your life, seek help immediately.

Treatment of depression starts with a frank discussion between you and your family about why you're depressed. The discussion should then involve your doctor. Treatment may consist of counseling, behavior modification, or psychiatric analysis. Antidepression drugs may be prescribed. The selective serotonin reuptake inhibitors (SSRIs)—Celexa, Paxil, Prozac, and Zoloft—are the most commonly prescribed antidepression drugs. They raise the levels serotonin in the brain. Low levels of serotonin are associated with

Table 2   Depression questionnaire

1. I feel sad.	Yes	No
2. I feel discouraged.	Yes	No
3. I feel blue.	Yes	No
4. I feel like I'm a failure.	Yes	No
5. I often feel isolated.	Yes	No
6. I feel sick.	Yes	No
7. I feel guilty.	Yes	No
8. I feel like I'm being punished.	Yes	No
9. I feel disappointed in myself.	Yes	No
10. I hate myself.	Yes	No
11. I blame myself for bad things that happen.	Yes	No
12. I cry a lot.	Yes	No
13. I feel irritable.	Yes	No
14. I don't care about what is happening around me.	Yes	No
15. I don't care about other people.	Yes	No
16. I can't make decisions.	Yes	No
17. I feel unattractive.	Yes	No
18. I can't work.	Yes	No
19. I can't fall asleep.	Yes	No
20. I can't stay awake.	Yes	No
21. I feel tired.	Yes	No
22. I have no appetite.	Yes	No
23. I don't care about sex.	Yes	No
24. I worry about everything.	Yes	No
25. I feel ashamed.	Yes	No

depression and anxiety. The SSRIs take at least 2 to 3 weeks to work. Side effects include fatigue, weight gain, and loss of sex drive, although they are less common in SSRIs than in other classes of anti-depression drugs. Wellbutrin increases brain dopamine levels in all regions of the brain, not just the ones that PD impacts. It is helpful in the apathetic depression of PD. Side effects include agitation and rarely seizures.

54. Will I lose my mind?

Approximately 30% of all people with PD develop a **dementia**, which is defined as a loss of previously acquired thinking skills. A mild loss of some of these skills is not dementia, but a marked loss of many of them is. Sometimes family members overlook changes in thinking and assume that the patient is exhibiting willful behavior or that the changes are part of a depression. Some patients are good at concealing their problems by deferring questions to other members of the family or by denying that there's a problem. It is important for your doctor to ask the patient and you, his family member, about changes in behavior, personality, or symptoms of confusion, fearfulness, disorientation, or withdrawal.

Dementia
a loss of previously acquired thinking skills.

PD dementia starts "silently," similar to PD itself. It also progresses slowly. PD dementia occurs in people who are 70 or more years old. Generally, a 10- to 15-year lag exists between PD and PD dementia. PD dementia results from a loss of nerve cells in different regions of the brain: The cells produce dopamine, norepinephrine, or acetylcholine. The dementia of PD is associated with

Lewy bodies, round structures inside the cell. It may be referred to as diffuse Lewy Body disease, diffuse Lewy Body dementia, Lewy Body disease, or Lewy Body dementia; depending on the specific region or regions affected and the degree to which they're affected, a variety of affective, behavioral, cognitive, and psychiatric symptoms appears. The time of appearance, the degree of severity, and the type and variety of symptoms usually, but not always, enables a doctor to distinguish one dementia from another.

Certain disorders may cause dementia-like symptoms, but if the cause is found and can be treated, the symptoms disappear. The more common dementia-like symptoms are as follows:

1. Depression consisting of apathy, indifference, and unwillingness to do or say anything may mimic dementia.
2. Kidney failure.
3. Liver failure.
4. Thyroid disease, either an underactive or an overactive gland.
5. Thiamine (vitamin B1) deficiency.
6. Vitamin B12 deficiency, which may result in anemia (called pernicious anemia), difficulty with balance, and real dementia.
7. A slow-growing tumor or a blood clot in a "silent region" of the brain—a region is where a tumor or blood clot can grow to a large size without initially causing headache or paralysis.

55. My husband "sees" people in our bedroom. What's happening?

Hallucinations may occur in people who are treated with PD drugs. They are usually visual and are often accompanied by delusions. The combination is called a **psychosis**. It may be difficult or even impossible for you to convince your spouse that there isn't anyone there or that you aren't going to harm him or her. Such symptoms cause distress to families and are the most frequently given reason for placing a patient in a nursing home.

Psychosis may occur without dementia as in LSD, amphetamine, or cocaine psychosis, and dementia may occur without psychosis as in LBD or **Alzheimer's disease**; however, in the presence of dementia, psychosis is more likely to appear. Symptoms of psychosis include **hallucinations,** seeing things that don't exist; **delusions,** a belief in something with no basis in reality; and **paranoia,** a belief that people are seeking to harm you. Obsessions with specific topics such as germs, sex, or death and dying, and compulsions such as gambling, eating, talking, and sex, are more common than reported.

When treated with PD drugs, PD patients, whether their dementia is recognized or unrecognized, can develop a psychosis that "unmasks" an underlying dementia. The type and severity of the psychosis will depend on the underlying dementia and the type and amount of the drugs. Anticholinergic drugs, such as Artane, Cogentin, Kemadrin and Symmetrel, are used in PD to control tremor; other anticholinergic drugs, Ditropan and Detrol, control bladder irritability; and still others, such as Elavil and Sinequan, are used to

Progression

Psychosis

a mental disorder in which delusions and hallucinations are combined; the person is convinced that unreal things or people truly exist.

Alzheimer's disease

a brain disorder characterized by memory loss and dementia. It is not related to Parkinson disease but has some similar symptoms.

Hallucinations

a delusion in which a person sees or hears things or people that don't exist.

Delusions

a belief in something with no basis in reality.

Paranoia

a belief that people are seeking to harm you.

treat depression or insomnia. Such drugs are more likely to cause psychosis than dopamine drugs. Among the dopamine drugs, the agonists Mirapex, Requip, and Permax are more likely to cause psychosis than Sinemet.

Psychosis may appear in people with PD who are not on anticholinergic drugs, agonists, or Sinemet. Although a psychosis may uncover an underlying dementia, it does not necessarily mean that a person has a dementia or will develop a dementia. A psychosis is reversible if the cause is found, but a dementia is not reversible.

The psychosis in PD resembles the psychosis in young people without dementia who overdose on drugs such as amphetamine, methamphetamine, cocaine, and ecstasy. It also resembles, in part, the psychosis of schizophrenia. The situations in PD in which psychosis may appear, other than after the addition of a new drug, are as follows:

- *Intensive care unit psychosis.* This occurs when a person with PD in an intensive care unit—with bells ringing, beepers beeping, lights flashing, and strangers coming and going—is sleep deprived and develops a psychosis. An underlying dementia may or may not exist.
- *Postoperative psychosis.* In this instance, a person with PD develops a psychosis after surgery and anesthesia, depending on the type and duration of the surgery and anesthesia, the severity of blood loss, and the type and amount of fluids given. An underlying dementia may or may not exist.

- *Sundown psychosis.* Here, a person with PD develops a psychosis at night when in strange surroundings. An underlying dementia usually exists.
- *The "DTs."* Psychosis sometimes occurs when a person is inadvertently and abruptly withdrawn from alcohol.

Other causes of psychosis can include:

- Dehydration.
- A high fever.
- Hypoglycemia.
- Infections (usually of the lung and bladder). These may or may not be associated with fever.
- Kidney failure.
- Lung disease. Difficulty breathing may result in lack of brain oxygen, retention of carbon dioxide, and changes in acid–base balance.
- Liver failure.
- Strokes (especially if they occur in specific regions).
- Thyroid disease (especially an overactive thyroid).

In PD, dementia symptoms result from a loss of dopamine, norepinephrine, serotonin, and acetylcholine cells in different brain regions. The type and severity of the symptom will depend on the type, the severity, and the location of the cell loss. In PD psychosis, symptoms result from excess dopamine and perhaps norepinephrine and serotonin in different brain regions. The type and severity of the symptoms also will depend on the duration and the amount of treatment with PD drugs. Not all PD patients have all symptoms. Sometimes, even though the differences outlined appear clear cut, they're not, as described here:

- In dementia, you lack awareness. You do not realize or recognize that anything is wrong. In psychosis, you are super or hyperaware of your surroundings.
- In dementia, you lack alertness. You sleep all day. In psychosis, you're awake all night, and you may or may not sleep during the day.
- In dementia, you have difficulty with memory. You can't remember the day, the date, the year, or where you are, and you get lost in a new place. In psychosis, your memory may be intact, but you may be so anxious and so distracted that you can't remember.
- In dementia, you have difficulty paying attention. You can't remember how to spell a word such as W-O-R-L-D backward. In psychosis, you can't pay attention long enough to spell W-O-R-L-D backward.
- In dementia, you have difficulty with calculations. You may be unable to balance your checkbook or make change. In psychosis, you may be unable to pay attention long enough to balance your checkbook or make change.
- In dementia, you have difficulty using and understanding words. You forget what certain words mean, and you can't think of the name of an object. In psychosis, you're too distracted to think.
- In dementia, you have difficulty following directions or instructions, as hard as you may try. You may be unable to organize, plan, or think of new ideas. In psychosis, you can't sit still long enough to do anything.
- In dementia, you may be apathetic and may take no interest in people or in your surroundings. You may appear depressed, but you're not. Usually you're not sad, and you don't feel guilty. In psychosis, your moods are inappropriate; for example, you're happy

when others are sad. You change rapidly and go from being down to up to down for no apparent reasons. You're very anxious and panic easily.

- In dementia, you may have obsessions and compulsions. You may have "passive" compulsions, humming or repeating stereotyped phrases. In psychosis, you may have "positive" but destructive obsessions and compulsions. You may be obsessed with germs to the exclusion of all activities, or you may have a compulsion to gamble, eat, collect trash, or engage in aberrant sexual behavior.
- In dementia, you are not able to read this. In psychosis, you are able to read this, but you would not.

56. Why am I obsessed?

Prior to the introduction of L-dopa, doctors described a "PD" personality: a person who was controlling, who had a need to do things "just so," who was obsessed with orderliness and cleanliness. Today this person might be diagnosed as having an obsessive–compulsive disorder (OCD). After the introduction of L-dopa there were reports of obsessive–compulsive behavior in many people with PD who were on L-dopa. The behavior included an obsessive fixation on sex. Indeed, at one time, L-dopa was thought to be an aphrodisiac (it is not). The behavior included an obsessive, excessive fixation on the patient's symptoms, and in some people, compulsive eating, compulsive gambling, compulsive praying, and compulsive shopping. Whether such behavior was present before L-dopa or was caused by L-dopa has never been resolved. The introduction of the dopamine agonists—first Parlodel, then Permax, then Mirapex, and then Requip—reignited the debate.

In the United States, 1 in 50 adults, about 5,000,000 people, are thought to have OCD (5 times as many people as have PD). Worries, doubts, and "magical" beliefs are common in everyday life. However, when they become excessive and dominate a person's life then a diagnosis of OCD is made. In OCD, it seems as though your brain gets stuck on a particular thought or urge and can't let go.

Obsessions are thoughts, images, or impulses that occur over and over again. You don't want them, you may find them disturbing, and you may realize they don't make sense, but they continue to dominate your life. Obsessions may be accompanied by feelings of fear, disgust, or doubt. If you have OCD you may try, subconsciously, to "divert" your mind from your obsessions by performing "rituals" or compulsions. Compulsions are acts you perform over and over again, often according to certain "rules." Thus you may repeatedly check to see if you have taken your pills. Many of the rituals give you no pleasure, but you do them because you are "compelled." Some of your compulsions, although you know they are destructive, give you pleasure. These include compulsive gambling, shopping, and compulsive sex, including pornography, phone sex, and video sex.

Obsessions and compulsions take up a lot of time and interfere with your work, social life, and family relationships. Most people with PD who are afflicted with obsessions and compulsions recognize at some point that these actions are unreasonable. If they don't recognize that these obsessive-compulsive beliefs and actions are unreasonable, this may suggest they are "incubating" a dementia.

Obsessions and compulsions can start at any time, from preschool age to adulthood. On average, people with obsessions and compulsions see three to four doctors and may spend many years seeking treatment before they are diagnosed. Obsessions and compulsions tend to be underdiagnosed because people with them may be secretive or lack insight about them. Research suggests that obsessions and compulsions involve problems in communication between your frontal-orbital and cingulate lobes and your basal ganglia. These brain structures use the chemical messengers dopamine and serotonin. It is believed that low levels of serotonin are prominently involved in obsessions and compulsions. High, and paradoxically low, levels of dopamine may also be involved. Drugs that increase the brain concentration of serotonin often improve obsessions and compulsions. Such drugs include the selective serotonin reuptake inhibitors, drugs such as Paxil, Prozac, and Zoloft, that are also used to treat depression.

There is no test for OCD. Rather, the diagnosis is made based on an assessment of the person's symptoms. A disorder associated with OCD is Tourette's Syndrome. Tourette's Syndrome is characterized by motor and vocal tic disorders. Tics are quick, involuntary, jerk-like movements. They include grimaces, shrugs, grunts and snorts. Tourette's is thought to result from high dopamine levels and resembles, in part, people with PD who have dyskinesia. Depression and OCD often occur together. Although stress can make

OCD worse, most people with OCD report that their symptoms may come and go unrelated to stress. People with OCD may abuse drugs. This may occur in some PD patients who become "addicted" to Sinemet, living for their next "on" and dreading their next "off."

57. What is the autonomic nervous system (ANS)?

Autonomic nervous system (ANS)

the region of the brain and nervous system that regulates the body's internal environment.

The **autonomic nervous system** (ANS), as its name implies, regulates the body's internal environment. The ANS is affected early in MSA and late in PD. If, originally, you did not have ANS symptoms, but they have appeared, this indicates PD has progressed: It has involved cells outside the substantia nigra.

Shortly after you arrive in a doctor's office or an emergency room, your vital signs are checked: temperature, pulse rate, blood pressure, and rate of respiration. The vital signs mirror your body's internal environment, which mirrors your ANS. Your ANS does the following:

- *Maintains your temperature at 98.6 Fahrenheit.* Your temperature rises because of an infection from bacteria, or a virus; an inflammation of a joint, a muscle, or a vein (phlebitis); a sauna, a steam bath, or a sun burn. Your ANS rids your body of heat by shuttling blood from your internal organs to your skin, and from here it radiates or evaporates. As a result you feel flushed or feverish. If you're anxious, your ANS can be subconsciously "tricked" into thinking your temperature's up (when it's not) and you may feel flushed or feverish. Your temperature drops because of an underactive thyroid gland, or a dip in the Arctic Ocean. Your ANS warms you by shuttling blood away from your skin to your internal organs. As a result, you may feel cold or turn blue. If you have PD, or if you're anxious, fearful, or panicked your ANS can be "tricked" into thinking your temperature's down (when it's not) and you may feel cold (when no one else does).

- *Maintains your pulse, or heart, rate between 60 to 90 beats/minute.* If your temperature, need for oxygen, or metabolism increases; if you lose body fluids (by dehydration or bleeding); or if you're in pain, then your ANS, through a "direct line" to your heart, can make it beat faster. If you have PD, or if you're anxious, your ANS can be "tricked" into making your heart beat faster and you may feel your heart pounding (or think it's pounding). Or you may feel dizzy, or lightheaded, or faint.

- *Maintains your blood pressure between 95–140/50–90.* To maintain a stabile internal environment, blood flow to critical organs must be adequate. Because flow cannot be easily measured, blood pressure is measured instead. The relationship is: Blood Pressure = Blood Flow Resistance of the Blood Vessels. Your tissues lose blood if your blood pressure falls when you stand up quickly, if you're dehydrated, or for other reasons. For flow to remain unchanged, the resistance of your vessels must increase. This is done by your ANS, which increases resistance by narrowing your arteries. If, despite the narrowing, blood pressure continues to drop, flow to critical organs, such as the brain, the heart, and the lungs, is maintained by shunting blood away from less critical organs such as the gut, the kidneys, the liver, or the skin. In this case, your ANS changes the resistance of your veins because 70% of circulating blood is in your veins. If you have PD, you are taking drugs for PD, or if you're anxious, fearful, or panicked, your ANS can be "tricked" into decreasing the resistance of your arteries or veins, dropping your blood pressure, and thereby making you feel dizzy, or lightheaded.

- *Maintains your respiratory rate below 18 breaths/minute.* This is the body's way of preventing hyperventilation. If your need for oxygen, or your temperature, or your metabolism rises, your ANS responds by making you breathe faster. As you do so, each breath is shallower and you spend more energy on the mechanics of breathing. This fatigues your chest muscles, the "bellows" for your lungs, making you gasp for air. If you have PD, or if you're anxious, fearful, or panicked, your ANS can be "tricked" into making you breathe faster or hyperventilate. When you hyperventilate, you "blow off" carbon dioxide. This, in turn, can make your heart pound, your vision blur, or your ears ring, or can make you feel dizzy, lightheaded, or faint.

Hypothalamus

a region in the brain that controls all the glands and the autonomic nervous system.

The ANS starts in a region called the **hypothalamus**, runs down the brainstem to the spinal cord, then travels through nerves to supply all the major organs and the blood vessels. The autonomic nervous system has two parts: the sympathetic nervous system and the para-sympathetic nervous system. Most organs are governed by the sympathetic nervous system through its control of the organ's blood supply. Some organs, the eye, the salivary glands, the heart, and the lungs are governed by the sympathetic and para-sympathetic nervous system. Activity of the sympathetic system widens the pupil. Activity of the para-sympathetic system narrows the pupil. Activity of the sympathetic system decreases saliva. Activity of the para-sympathetic system increases saliva. Activity of the sympathetic system speeds up the heart. Activity of the para-sympathetic system slows the heart. Activity of the sympathetic system widens the airway- and improves breathing. Activity of the para-sympathetic system narrows the airway and causes wheezing. The ANS is asked to mobilize your body's defenses against fever, dehydration, pain, shock, anxiety, fear, terror, or panic. To prepare your body, for "flight, fright, or fight." The ANS is altered in PD and may not react as promptly or as appropriately as it should.

58. Can I black out from PD?

On February 1, 2002, Janet Reno, the former Attorney General of the United States, blacked out. Ms. Reno was giving a speech. She had been standing and talking for 45 minutes, she felt hot, and (as captured on television), she fell to the floor. She was immediately awakened, taken to a nearby hospital, evaluated overnight, and released the next day. Earlier, in 1998, while standing in church, Ms. Reno blacked out. The blackout occurred after Ms. Reno had completed a strenuous hike. A concern has been raised is that Ms. Reno, who is 63 years of age and has had PD for 6 years, blacked out because of her PD, or because of the drugs she's taking for PD, a dopamine agonist and Sinemet.

People with PD can black out. This is uncommon but does occur. The cause of the blackout is a decrease in blood flow to the brain. This occurs when a person with PD abruptly arises from a lying to a sitting or standing position. When you lie down, your heart and your head are at the same level. It is relatively easy for your heart, an electrically driven pump, to pump blood to your brain through the great arteries in the neck. When you go from a lying down to a sitting or standing position, your head is not higher than your heart, and your heart must now pump against gravity, working harder to pump blood to your brain. In order to maintain the same blood flow to your brain your body has three options: (1) Your ANS can make your heart beat faster. (2) Your ANS can increase the force of your heart's contractions so your heart can pump harder. (3) Your ANS can increase the resistance of the great arteries in your neck, so that the arteries contract. In some people with PD, the ANS is not as responsive, and thus when some people with PD stand up from a lying or sitting position, the blood pressure drops, the great arteries in the neck do not constrict or tighten, blood flow decreases to the brain, and the person blacks out. Certain drugs, including the dopamine agonists, can exacerbate this tendency.

Janet Reno did not black out because of PD. In the times she passed out, she was standing, not arising from a lying or sitting to a standing position, so she did not experience the type of black-out that is experienced by some people with PD. Blacking out while standing for a long period of time in one place (more than 30 minutes) occurs for different reasons than blacking out while arising from a lying or sitting to a standing position. If you stand long enough in one place—30 minutes is long enough in some people—then blood pools in the veins and capillaries of your feet. Such blood is not available to be carried through the great veins into the filling chambers of the heart. A decrease in the blood flowing into the filling chambers of the heart results in a decrease in the pumping actions of the emptying chambers of the heart (they need a certain volume of blood to operate efficiently), this results in a drop in blood pressure, followed by a decrease in the flow of blood to the brain, and this results in a blackout. A person can be perfectly healthy, but can black out if he or she stands for a long period of time they. Thus Army or Marine recruits who stand at "parade rest" for long periods of time can, and do, black out. The factors increasing the tendency to black out while standing as distinct from rising from a lying to a standing position are: (1) The length of time you stand. You are more likely to black out standing for 45 minutes (as Ms. Reno did) than standing for 30 minutes. (2) Whether the place where you are standing is very warm or hot. If the place is hot you perspire, and can become dehydrated, which results in even less fluid being returned to the filling chambers of the heart. This contributed to Ms. Reno's recent blackout while speaking, and to her 1997 blackout. If you are going to be in a warm place where you will perspire, be certain to drink a lot of water. (3) The presence of other factors that could result in dehydration, such as a virus. (4) The presence of varicose veins. Varicose veins permit increased pooling of blood in the veins of the feet and legs making less available for the filling chambers of the heart. If you have varicose veins, wearing elastic stockings can help prevent black-outs by "toning" the veins.

59. Does shortness of breath mean I'm worse?

Breathing is a basic function that occurs automatically, usually without conscious awareness. Breathing is controlled by the respiratory center in the brainstem. When a signal arrives from the respiratory center, the chest wall muscles and the diaphragm contract. This increases the space between the chest wall and the lungs, which in turn decreases the pressure inside the lungs. The lungs inhale to equalize the pressure inside with the pressure outside. As the lungs expand to fill the space in the chest wall, a second signal is sent to relax the muscles. The brainstem makes its decisions regarding the rate and depth of breathing on the basis of information it receives from the body. This information includes the level of oxygen in the air, the level of oxygen in the blood, the level of expired gas (carbon dioxide) in the blood, and the acidity or alkalinity of the blood. The carbon dioxide level is the single most critical factor for controlling the rate and depth of breathing because the carbon dioxide level reflects the rate of energy consumption.

Shortness of breath, difficulty breathing, or a conscious awareness of breathing can occur because of disease of the heart. The heart is a muscle, a pump, that circulates fluid through the body. If the heart muscle is damaged by repeated heart attacks, by inflammation, or by drugs such as alcohol, the pump fails and fluid (edema) accumulates in the lungs. If you are having shortness of breath, have your heart checked.

Shortness of breath occurs because of interference with air flow through the nose, the trachea (the windpipe) or the bronchi (the airways). The interference can be caused by inflammation, infection, or obstruction of the nose or airways. Shortness of breath occurs because of interference with the exchange of oxygen from the air to the lungs. By interfering with the flow of air into the lungs or with the exchange of oxygen, a person works harder to breathe, decreasing the amount of oxygen absorbed with each breath and the amount of waste gas (carbon dioxide) exhaled with each breath. Risk factors for lung disease include (1) Cigarette smoking (a major risk), including marijuana smoking; (2) occupations where chemicals or dusts are chronically inhaled such as occurs in asbestos workers, coal miners, or firemen; (3) chronic infections such as tuberculosis.

Shortness of breath can occur after mild exertion or exercise that previously did not result in shortness of breath. Or the shortness of breath can occur after lying down. The circumstances in which the shortness of breath occurs may indicate whether the shortness of breath results from heart or lung disease. Thus shortness of breath after lying down is more likely to indicate fluid backing up from a failing heart than from a failing lung. Shortness of breath from a failing lung (known as emphysema) is more likely to occur with exertion or exercise. Coughing and wheezing may accompany shortness of breath with both lung and heart disease.

Shortness of breath occurs in diseases that weaken the muscles of the chest wall and diaphragm. These are the muscles that surround the lungs and act as a bellows. During inspiration they contract, dropping the pressure around the lungs, which causes the lungs to expand, forcing air from the atmosphere into the alveoli. During expiration the chest wall muscles relax, narrowing the space around the lungs and expelling air. Diseases that cause weakness of the muscles of the chest wall and diaphragm include muscular dystrophy, myasthenia gravis, and Lou Gehrig's disease. The resulting paralysis is similar to the deliberate paralysis caused by curare-like agents that are used in anesthesia.

Shortness of breath in PD can occur in several ways:

- The chest wall muscles and diaphragm can become rigid. During inspiration they do not expand fully, and during expiration they do not relax fully. Thus, the bellows function of the lungs is compromised. At rest, the normal rate of breathing is 12 to 18 breaths per minute. In some patients with advanced Parkinson disease the rate is greater than 18 breaths per minute. The patients spend more energy breathing, fatigue more easily, and become short of breath. If they also have heart or lung disease, or a history of smoking, these conditions will add to their shortness of breath.

- A severe deformity of the spine can occur, restricting the movement of the lungs and resulting in shortness of breath. While some Parkinson patients have a mild degree of deformity, it's the rare patient who has a deformity of sufficient severity to cause shortness of breath. Such patients are more comfortable sitting or standing than lying down.

- Dyskinesia can occur. Some people who fluctuate—who have "on" and "off" periods on levodopa—may complain of shortness of breath. The shortness of breath can occur when they're "off," before they take their levodopa, when their chest wall muscles and diaphragm are rigid. Or the shortness of breath can occur when they're "on" when they have dyskinesia, because it may cause the chest wall muscles and diaphragm to contract less efficiently. People with PD with rigid chest walls, severe spinal deformities, or severe "off" periods may complain of shortness of breath with exertion or exercise. Sometimes they may complain of shortness of breath when lying down. Normally, if you sit or stand gravity aids the downward movement of the diaphragm. If you lay down, you lose the aid of gravity. Some people with PD are unable to compensate for this loss, and complain of shortness of breath. In some people the shortness of breath is so bothersome they are encouraged to sleep sitting up in a chair.

- People with PD, like anyone else, can be anxious, which can result in shortness of breath.

If a person with PD complains of shortness of breath, either on exertion or lying down this must be evaluated. Proper diagnosis may require an internist, a cardiologist, and a lung specialist. If the shortness of breath is not related to heart or lung disease, or if contributing factors can be ruled out, then it's probable the shortness of breath is related to PD. Shortness of breath means your PD has progressed, and that the muscles of the chest wall are involved now. But it does not mean you will die! If the shortness of breath is related to rigidity of the chest wall muscles and diaphragm, additional PD drugs—especially a long-acting dopamine agonist such as Mirapex or Requip—may help. If the shortness of breath is related to dyskinesia, then levodopa should be reduced. To compensate for the reduced levodopa, a long-acting agonist such as Mirapex or Requip can be added.

60. I can't swallow. Is this PD?

Depending on how the question is asked, 30% to 95% of people with PD say they have difficulty swallowing. In most, the difficulty is minor, but in some it's major.

Swallowing requires the coordinated action of many muscles, both voluntary and smooth. First, your tongue and jaw muscles prepare the food to be swallowed by chewing it and mixing it with saliva. Then, the muscles in the back of your mouth and throat start the swallow. They also seal off your windpipe and nose to keep food and liquids from backing up into them. Next, the muscles of your esophagus propel the food into your stomach. Slow or rigid muscles, at any level, can result in difficulty swallowing. The same slowness and rigidity that affects the muscles in your arms and legs affects the muscles in your throat. A serious complication of difficulty swallowing is aspiration pneumonia. About 25% of people with PD aspirate at one time or another. In many, aspiration is announced by coughing or choking. In some, it's "silent." Difficulty swallowing may result in marked and unintentional weight loss.

Treating the primary symptoms of PD—rigidity and slowness—by increasing or adjusting Sinemet plus Comtan, the dopamine agonists, or the anticholinergic drugs is helpful in 50% of people. Detrol, which is helpful in treating drooling, may also be helpful in swallowing. Training sessions with speech and swallowing therapists are also helpful. In a small group of people with PD, perhaps 5%, abnormal muscle bands may partly block swallowing, or pouches may form, trapping food. In these people, identified by a barium swallow test, surgery may correct the difficulty.

If you have difficulty swallowing, complete the *Swallowing Questionnaire* and discuss it with your doctor.

1. I've lost weight recently.	Yes	No
2. I drool.	Yes	No
3. I cough when I eat or drink.	Yes	No

4. I choke when I eat or drink.	Yes	No
5. I have heartburn.	Yes	No
6. I have difficulty propelling food to the back of my mouth.	Yes	No
7. I have difficulty keeping food or liquids in my mouth.	Yes	No
8. It takes me a long time to finish eating.	Yes	No
9. Food sticks in my throat.	Yes	No
10. I have difficulty swallowing pills.	Yes	No

The following advice from Dr. Robert Pfeiffer may improve your swallowing. Take small bites. Swallow twice after every bite. Take small sips. Alternate bites and sips. This clears the food from your mouth. Don't talk with food in your mouth. Keep your chin parallel to the table. If your chin's too far down, you can't keep food in your mouth. If your chin's too far up, this opens up your windpipe, increasing your risk of aspiration. People with PD may, without knowing it, bend their necks, forcing their chins down. This makes chewing (and swallowing) difficult. Bend your neck so your eyes look at the floor. Now try to chew. It's difficult because by bending your neck you put your jaw muscles at a mechanical disadvantage. Now raise your neck so your eyes look 30 degrees above the horizontal. Now try to chew. It's easy because your jaw muscles are at a mechanical advantage. Because you can't always remind yourself to raise your chin, I tell people with PD to sit with their elbows on the table, which automatically raises their chin and helps chewing and swallowing. Finally, you can change your diet. Certain foods such as raw vegetables, nuts, and peanut butter may be difficult to swallow and should be avoided. A swallowing therapist or a dietitian can recommend foods that are easy to swallow.

61. Why do I drool?

Drooling (sialorrhea) results from difficulty in swallowing. Most of the time drooling is an annoyance. However, sometimes it's an embarrassment, and sometimes it's even a hazard: Aspiration of saliva (swallowing saliva into your lungs) may result in pneumonia. Swallowing requires coordination of the muscles of your lips, tongue, mouth, and throat. Gravity aids in swallowing. During the day, when your head is erect (while you're seated or standing), saliva, propelled by your tongue, palate, and throat, moves down your esophagus into your stomach. In PD, the muscles of your tongue, palate, throat, and esophagus may be affected. The muscles become rigid and slow and lose their ability to propel food downward. This usually (but not always) occurs at a late stage in PD. Anything that impairs your ability to swallow food also impairs your ability to swallow saliva. Saliva is produced by glands located in the floor of your mouth at the angle of the jaw. Although the production of saliva is automatic, its production can be increased in response to external events. Thus, the sight, smell, or taste of food (even the thought of food) increases the flow of saliva. The ANS controls the production of saliva. Early in PD, you may experience difficulty in swallowing saliva as wetness of your pillow. During the day, with your head upright, gravity compensates for any difficulty in swallowing saliva. At night, with your head down, gravity no longer compensates—and saliva drips onto your pillow.

The first approach to treating drooling is educational. The reasons for drooling are explained: You are taught to sleep with your head upright and to chew food slowly and carefully, swallowing frequently. These suggestions help, but eventually, as PD progresses, this is not enough. The next approach is to prescribe anticholinergic drugs, which block the actions of acetylcholine at **cholinergic receptors** on the salivary glands. Artane and Cogentin block the actions of acetylcholine on receptors on the salivary gland, thus decreasing drooling; however, few PD patients can tolerate the high doses of Artane or Cogentin required to control drooling without side effects. Atropine, in solution and in small doses, taken as drops three to four times a day, may help. Such solutions have fewer side effects than Artane and Cogentin.

Cholinergic receptors

proteins on cells to which molecules of acetylcholine attach.

62. I'm constipated. Is this PD?

Constipation is frequent in PD. Not having a daily bowel movement isn't constipation. In fact, three bowel movements per week is normal. Constipation is defined as two or less bowel movements per week. In studying constipation, doctors measure the "colon transit time," which is twice as long in people with PD, with or without constipation, as in comparably aged people. Decreased frequency of bowel movements, two per less per week, occurs in 30% of people with PD. However, difficulty completing a bowel movement, with straining and incomplete evacuation, called difficulty defecating, is more common, occurring in 70% of people with PD. Many people have both constipation and difficulty defecating, and it's important to distinguish between them because their treatments differ.

In some people with PD (perhaps 5%), constipation and difficulty defecating result in fecal impaction, bloating, discomfort, and pain. A rectal examination diagnoses constipation. Usually, the impaction has to be removed manually. Proper bowel habits can prevent impaction.

Normally, the muscles of your bowel wall propel your stool forward; however, the rigidity and slowness that affects other muscles can affect your bowels. Because the bowels move slowly, stool moves slowly, and the fluid that's mixed in with the stool dries out, making the stools hard. The longer that the stool takes to pass through the bowel, the harder it becomes, and the more difficult it becomes to pass. The ANS and the bowel's own nervous system, the **enteric nervous system**, a cousin to the ANS, help to regulate bowels.

Enteric nervous system

the nervous system that regulates the bowels.

To defecate, the muscles of your belly must squeeze down, and the muscles of your pelvis must relax. The muscles encircling your colon and anus must squeeze out your stool, and your anal sphincter must open. A lack of coordination among these muscles coupled with rigidity and slowness results in difficulty defecating. Before assuming that your difficulty results from PD, conditions such as polyps, tumors, and diverticulitis must be excluded. An evaluation should include a rectal exam, a proctoscopy, or sigmoidoscopy, and if necessary, a colonoscopy.

As your colon transit time slows, water is absorbed from your stool, making it hard. Fiber, in addition to "cleansing" your bowel, acts like sawdust soaking up water, allowing it to remain in your stool, preventing your stool from drying out and becoming hard. In a study in which dietary fiber intake was estimated in people with PD, it was found that the average fiber intake was only two thirds of the recommended daily dose of 20 grams. Increased dietary fiber then is the first step and is achieved by eating fiber-rich foods such as fruits, including dates, figs, and prunes, vegetables, unprocessed bran cereal, whole grains, and beans such as fava and kidney beans. Dietary fiber can be supplemented with methyl cellulose (Citrucel), psyllium (Metamucil), or polycarbophil (FiberCon or Fiberall). With this approach, you should drink six to eight glasses of water a day. All of these can be supplemented with a stool softener such as Colace.

Regular exercise to strengthen the muscles of your abdomen and pelvis is helpful. Walking promotes movement of stool into your colon and rectum. A laxative should be avoided but may be used if the previously mentioned measures fail. Start with lactulose, or sorbital, or GoLytely, a glycol solution, used to clean the bowels before colonoscopy. Enemas or "irritant laxatives" such as bisacodyl, cascara, or magnesia are last resorts.

Treatment for constipation may not help defecation and may sometimes make things worse by increasing your need to have a bowel movement without improving your ability to do so. Evidence exists that people with PD when they're off (when Sinemet isn't working) have more difficulty with constipation.

63. I urinate all the time. Why?

The normal process of bladder filling proceeds in silence as your bladder's walls become distended. You're not conscious of this until the contents of your bladder reach approximately 1,000 ml (1 liter). At this point, your bladder starts signaling your brain that the time for emptying has arrived. Your brain—consciously now—keeps your bladder from emptying until you find a suitable place to void. Once all is ready, your brain gives the "go signal." Your bladder contracts while at the same time a system of sphincters that have kept your bladder closed relaxes.

In PD, malfunction in the basal ganglia results in a bladder that contracts prematurely at low amounts of urine, lower than 1,000 ml. Such premature contractions are not strong enough to make your bladder to empty; however, they generate enough signals to create an urge to void. You rush to the bathroom only to empty a small amount of urine. As the process repeats itself, the trips to the bathroom become more frequent. Urgency can be so strong that if you don't reach a bathroom on time, you have an "accident."

If this happens, see a urologist, who will ask you to void and will do a urine analysis to exclude bleeding, an infection, or diabetes. After you void, he or she may place a catheter inside your bladder to determine whether you have completely emptied it. If you retain 100 ml of urine in your bladder, you are at risk for infections. The urologist will then do a rectal examination to check the size of your prostate. Then the urologist will use a "scope" to see whether your bladder's inflamed or if there's a tumor. If you're a woman, the urologist will see whether your bladder neck's narrowed. Based on this evaluation, and a series of tests called "urodynamics," the urologist may prescribe drugs to "relax" the muscles of your bladder.

One drug, Detrol LA, blocks receptors for acetylcholine along the bladder wall. The cholinergic receptors in the bladder are a special class called **muscarinic**

receptors. Detrol LA (long acting) is a newer antimuscarinic taken once daily; it has a smoother and longer duration of action than its predecessor, Detrol (tolterodine tartrate). Detrol LA has a relatively weak action on cholinergic receptors outside of the bladder. This is important because drugs that block cholinergic receptors outside of the bladder can result in side effects. Although such side effects may occur with Detrol LA, they're less common. Another drug, Ditropan, is an anticholinergic drug. It blocks a set of nerves, the cholinergic nerves, that carry impulses to the bladder's muscle and internal sphincter. Side effects of anticholinergic drugs include dryness of mouth, aggravation of glaucoma, and constipation.

Incontinence may be related to urgency and frequency. It may be a separate condition. Embarrassment is the main reason incontinence is not discussed. Even your doctor may feel embarrassed bringing it up. Incontinence, involuntary loss of urine, may lead to decreased self-esteem and to withdrawal from social activities. It could be that PD slows your ability to get to the bathroom, or to undo your clothes. In women who have had children, incontinence may be related to weakness of the pelvic muscles. Incontinence in women can be treated with Detrol LA, with special strengthening procedures called Kegel exercises. Sometimes surgery is needed. In men, an enlarged prostrate, may cause incontinence.

In PD there are different kinds of bladder dysfunction all of which can lead to incontinence. The causes include an overactive bladder, an underactive bladder, an overactive sphincter, an underactive sphincter, and a sphincter not synchronized to your bladder. Through an examination, including "urodynamics," a urologist can determine where the problem is and how to treat it.

Muscarinic receptors

cholinergic receptors in the bladder.

Progression

Drugs, exercise, and surgery aside, there are common sense ways to deal with incontinence. If nighttime incontinence is a problem because it's hard to get out of bed, keeping a urinal or a commode next to your bed is a solution. There are pads to protect your bed and plastic sheets to protect your mattress. Most supermarkets carry a line of pads and protective undergarments for incontinence. These pads have a special absorbent core that holds the urine, shielding it from your skin. They also help to prevent urine odor. No PD patient should be inhibited by incontinence.

64. I can't get an erection. Why?

Few men bring up this issue with their doctors, and few doctors ask about it. This doesn't mean it's unimportant. The ability to achieve and maintain an erection is frustrating, embarrassing, and distressing to you and your partner. Achieving and maintaining an erection results from the successful interplay of several different physical and psychological processes. One or more of these may be impaired in PD. Thus, anxiety and or depression may result in a loss of a desire to have or think about sex. The desire to have sex or think about sex is called libido. A loss of libido results in impotence. Most men with PD, however, retain their desire for sex, and this coupled with impotence, heightens frustration, results in abstinence, and deepens social isolation.

PD usually begins at age 60, a time when many men experience impotence related to vascular disease, diabetes, an enlarged prostrate, or depression. Thus, impotence should not automatically be attributed to PD. Diabetes, an underactive or overactive thyroid, adrenal, or pituitary gland, or a deficiency of testosterone may cause impotence. Disease of the arteries and veins may cause impotence. Smoking, diabetes, high blood pressure, and high cholesterol promote disease of the arteries. Men with arterial disease may have difficulty in attaining an erection, whereas men with disease of the veins may have difficulty in maintaining an erection. Disease of the veins results in impotence because the veins are unable to constrict. After an erection is attained, blood normally leaks from the penis back into the veins, causing the penis to soften. After an erection is attained, the veins constrict, preventing leakage of blood from the penis maintaining the erection.

Some features of your appearance such as tremor may cause you to lose self-esteem. Other features such as drooling may make you think that you're unattractive to your partner. These features, if relevant, must be discussed and resolved. Some men (and women) because of their physical limitations no longer maintain proper grooming. Thus, hair may grow from their nose or ears, or their teeth may be dirty. If relevant, these features should be remedied. Some people because they move slowly and cannot turn in bed become unduly anxious and cannot perform sexually. For them, taking Sinemet or a dopamine agonist (Mirapex, Requip) an hour before intercourse is helpful.

Alcohol, in moderation (because it represses social inhibitions), may promote sexual activity. In excess, alcohol depresses the brain and can temporarily result in impotence. Antihistamines, cocaine, marijuana, major tranquilizers, sedatives, and some anti-depression drugs may aggravate or cause impotence by depressing the brain. Some of these drugs may block ejaculation. Some drugs that lower high blood pressure may cause impotence. This may be related to the drop in blood pressure. Drugs that regulate blood pressure by regulating the ANS are more likely to cause impotence. The commonly used PD drugs rarely cause impotence. Impotence associated with their use invariably results from PD. As a rule, if impotence occurs within a few days or a month of starting a drug, the drug should be considered to be a potential cause of the impotence. If a drug aggravates or causes impotence, stopping the drug restores potency.

In PD, the main cause of impotence is ANS insufficiency. Impotence is usually, but not always, associated with other symptoms of ANS insufficiency. The ANS sends messages to the lower spinal cord, the parts involved in sexual function. The lower spinal cord sends messages through nerves to the penis and testes. If you are able to achieve and maintain an erection, this reflects adequate blood flow through the arteries to the penis, with appropriate filling and hardening of the penis. If you are unable to achieve or maintain an erection, this reflects a failure of the ANS system to constrict the veins surrounding the penis, resulting in softening.

Impotence must be acknowledged. You, or your partner, must bring up the issue and want to resolve it. Many men are reluctant to admit that they are impotent. If they do confess impotence, they do it at the end of their consultation—as an afterthought. This reflects their ambiguity and leaves no time for a frank discussion of a sensitive problem. If impotence is important, it alone should be the subject of your doctor's visit, and both you and your partner should attend. If discussing impotence in the presence of your partner is difficult, then you should go alone. You and your partner should recognize that your inability to talk as a couple may be part of the problem. Some men become obsessed with impotence. This, when it becomes all encompassing, can turn off even a sympathetic partner. The main ingredients to success in treating impotence are a willingness to seek help, to discuss everything openly, and to respect each other's needs.

Keep in mind that desire precedes arousal. Your partner should be aware of the problems that are unique to you. This includes a decreased sense of smell, resulting in an inability to be aroused by provocative odors, including perfumes, hair lotions, and body parts. Visual stimuli may be better: anything that works. Viagra, taken orally, is a potent blocker of an enzyme in the penis. Viagra increases the concentration of a naturally occurring compound, nitrous oxide, which allows blood to enter the penis. Studies indicate that Viagra is effective in many men with PD. Because blood pressure in PD patients may drop upon standing, you must consult with your doctor before using Viagra.

65. I have oily skin. Is this PD?

In some people, patches of oily, greasy, scaly, inflamed, reddened, and itchy skin develop in response to excess sebum production. Your scalp, the sides of your nose, your eyebrows, your eyelids, the skin behind your ears and the middle of your chest are the most common sites. These areas have the highest concentration of sebaceous glands. Associated with the dermatitis, dandruff may appear as scaling on your scalp without redness. Seborrheic dermatitis is common in infants, where it is called "cradle cap." Cradle cap usually clears without treatment by the age of 8 to 12 months. This may be related to the gradual disappearance of certain hormones that are passed from the mother to the child. Seborrheic dermatitis occurs in teen-agers where it is associated with acne or psoriasis. Seborrheic dermatitis occurs in older people and in people with PD. People recovering from stressful conditions, such as a heart attack, may also develop seborrheic dermatitis. In all of these conditions a combination of hormonal changes and a faulty ANS may be responsible for the excess sebum production. The condition is best treated by a dermatologist.

66. I think my PD is worse. What do I do?

It is not usual for PD to "suddenly" get worse. Because the progression of PD is slow, changes are barely perceptible and a "sudden" change is probably is not a result of the PD. Several things should be checked before you assume that it is the PD. First, have you missed any doses of medicine? If things have been going smoothly, it is sometimes easy to miss a dose and not have any noticeable effect. Over time, those missed doses will make a difference. When do you take your medications? Are the doses given at regular times of the day? The timing of doses is important. Sometimes a patient or caregiver will not understand the need for sequential doses throughout the day, thinking that it is the total amount of medication that is important. A problem could arise if another medication is interfering with your PD drugs. For instance, you may not take your early-morning dose of Sinemet because you have been advised to take Fosamax an hour before breakfast and on an empty stomach. If you delay taking Sinemet and take it at breakfast, your morning symptoms of PD will be worse. Taking levodopa with food or milk can also reduce its effectiveness. Before carbidopa was added to levodopa, many patients taking levodopa alone experienced nausea so that it became a common practice to advise them to take levodopa with food. The addition of carbidopa eliminated the nausea and made it possible to achieve better relief of symptoms from a smaller dose of levodopa. A lack of sleep or depression can also aggravate the symptoms of PD.

If none of these are happening, then you should look for an infection. Bladder infections or upper respiratory infections are the most likely culprits. It is likely that any of these situations can cause a temporary worsening of your symptoms without implying that there has been progression of your PD. Sometimes, changing the times when you take your drugs, clearing up a bladder infection, or simply getting enough sleep can relieve the problems.

PART SIX

Surgery for PD

Is there surgery for PD?

What is a thalamotomy?

What is pallidotomy?

More ...

67. Is there surgery for PD?

Surgery for PD and other movement disorders was pioneered in the 1940s by Meyers (United States). Large regions of the brain were exposed and using surface landmarks (there were no CT scans or MRIs) the basal ganglia—a series of interconnected regions of the brain including the striatum, globus pallidus, and thalamus—were located and ablated (destroyed). In 1947, Spiegel and Wycis developed a crown-like stereotaxic frame that held the head in place and allowed regions inside the brain to be correlated with reference points on the frame. In the 1950s Leksell (Sweden) pioneered pallidotomy for tremor. Later, in the late 1950s and 1960s Cooper (United States) and Narabayashi (Japan) pioneered thalamotomy for tremor. The introduction of levodopa dramatically reduced the need for surgery. Laitinen (Sweden) and De Long (United States) however, revived surgery by demonstrating the effectiveness of pallidotomy for levodopa-induced dyskinesias. Benebid (France) pioneered DBS of the STN. Lozano (Canada), Lang (Canada),and Koller (United States) refined DBS for PD and ET. All of these pioneers dramatically increased our understanding of the brain's anatomy, circuitry, and its effects on movement. Currently three types of surgery are performed: (1) **ablative** or destructive surgery; (2) stimulation surgery or deep brain stimulation (DBS); and (3) transplantation or restorative surgery.

Ablative procedures

procedures that destroy damaged tissues through ablation, or destruction using heat sources.

Ablative or destructive surgery refers to locating, targeting, then ablating or destroying a specific, clearly defined brain area or region. The area chosen is usually an area or region that's been altered or changed by PD, or a region that generates or produces an aberrant or abnormal chemical or electrical discharge. An abnormal discharge that in turn produces or generates an abnormal signal or "static." The static, in turn, interrupts the normal, harmonious operation of the brain. Destruction of the abnormal discharging brain region lessens or negates the static. This allows restoration of more normal or closer to normal function. Destruction of the abnormal discharging region rarely results in restoration of completely normal function.

Why doesn't destruction of the abnormal discharging region restore normal function? The brain is more than a circuit board. There's more wrong in PD than one abnormal discharging region. Only part of the abnormal discharging region may have been destroyed and, at a later date, the surgeon may have to operate again. To understand why only part of the abnormal discharging region may be destroyed requires understanding of the surgical procedure.

To ablate or destroy the abnormal discharging region, the surgeon heats the exploring probe or electrode—this coagulates, denatures, destroys the abnormal region. As the patient's awake during surgery, the surgeon can monitor the extent of the ablation by observing the patient's response. As an example, a patient with a left-hand tremor has the probe inserted into his brain's right side. The brain's right side controls the body's left side and vice-versa. The surgeon then heats, coagulates, and destroys part of the patient's right-thalamus, the abnormal discharging region. The abnormal electrical discharge is monitored through the probe—the same probe that later heats, coagulates, and destroys the abnormal region. When the patient's tremor ceases, the probe is removed.

Heating causes the surrounding thalamus to swell. Initially, the heat-induced swelling inactivates a larger, wider region than required to stop the tremor. After several days, or weeks, the heat-induced swelling subsides. Part of the thalamus remains quiet, no longer discharging. But part may recover, and the tremor may return. As an example, if you burn your hand—the equivalent of heating the thalamus—the swelling of your hand peaks in 48–96 hours, then subsides. The full extent of the burn, the size of the burn-induced scar won't be known for days or weeks, until the burn-induced swelling subsides. Most of the burn-induced swelling of the hand is temporary. Initially, however, the swelling masks the size of the underlying scar—which is permanent. Similarly when the thalamus is heated the size of the permanent scar is usually less than the initial swelling. Few surgeons can correctly estimate the size and intensity of the burn needed to permanently abolish a tremor. It's safer to induce a smaller burn—that is, to destroy a smaller region—and chance the tremor returning than to destroy a larger region and risk paralysis.

The surgery—ablative, destructive surgery and stimulation surgery, DBS—is painless. The scalp, which contains pain-sensitive nerves, is numbed with a local anesthetic. Next, a small hole is drilled into the skull. The skull and underlying brain covering, the dura, contain pain-sensitive nerves. They too are numbed with a local anesthetic. The brain itself contains no pain-sensitive nerves. The brain, especially the thalamus, receives, interprets, and causes the body to react to painful stimuli. However, because the brain itself contains no pain-sensitive nerves, it feels no pain. Ablative or destructive surgery doesn't cure PD. A troubling symptom—tremor, dyskinesia—may be removed, but PD isn't. PD is an inexorably progressive disease, and other symptoms eventually appear.

How many people go for surgery—all surgery? It's estimated there are 1 million PD patients in the United States. Fewer than 1,000 of PD patients (less than 0.1%) undergo surgery each year. Why so few? Because the surgery isn't for newly diagnosed patients, patients doing well on drugs (with the exception of tremor), patients with advanced disease who aren't responding to drugs, or patients with hallucinations, confusion, or memory loss. It's also not performed on patients who are hesitant or afraid. As surgery is improved and perfected, as it becomes safer, as new techniques and strategies are innovated, developed, and applied—a larger number of patients will opt for and benefit from surgery.

68. What is a thalamotomy?

Tremor probably results from "static" in a loop involving nerve cells in different parts of the brain, similar to "static" in a radio. The loop goes from the **cerebral cortex** to the striatum to the globus pallidus to the ventral lateral thalamus and then back to the cortex. Interrupting this circuit in the thalamus by means of a lesion, a **thalamotomy**, stops the tremor. The surgery is performed using a stereotaxic frame and MRI or CT scans to guide the surgeon in the placement of the lesion. The patient is sedated lightly, and a local analgesic is given for drilling through the skull. An microelectrode is passed through the brain to the target in

Cerebral cortex
the conscious, thinking brain.

Thalamotomy
a surgical procedure targeting the thalamus designed to stop tremors.

the thalamus. A test lesion is tried before placement of the permanent lesion. The lesion is made by a specific radio frequency current, which raises the temperature of the tip of the microelectrode and destroys a tiny section of the thalamus. The lesion is placed on the side of the brain opposite the side of the body affected, so if the left arm and left hand have the tremor, the lesion will be in the right thalamus. Thalamotomy done on both sides of the brain simultaneously may result in difficulty speaking or difficulty in balancing (loss of righting reflexes). Bilateral simultaneous thalamotomy is *not* recommended. The ideal person for thalamotomy has a tremor on only one side of his body, one that does not respond well to drugs. The person should be in good health without mental or psychiatric disorders. Thalamotomy can relieve tremor and rigidity, but it does not help bradykinesia or balance problems.

69. What is pallidotomy?

Pallidotomy

a surgical procedure that can decrease dyskinesia, reduce tremor, and improve bradykinesia by "releasing a brake" in the globus pallidus.

Pallidotomy is a surgical procedure that can decrease dyskinesia, reduce tremor, and improve bradykinesia. The ideal candidate is a young person who is healthy with no impairment in thinking and memory. The person should have a good response to PD drugs. This is unlike thalamotomy, where a good response to drugs is *not* necessary. Remember, tremor may *not* respond to PD drugs, while bradykinesia does, and dyskinesia results from PD drugs (levodopa). Pallidotomy is similar to thalamotomy except the target region is the globus pallidus. This region of the brain is known to be overactive in animal models of PD. The interruption of the outflow from the globus pallidus inhibits (blocks) the pathway that causes dyskinesias. The interruption of the outflow from the globus pallidus also "releases" a brake that blocks the substantia nigra. The results of pallidotomy on reducing dyskinesia, reducing tremor, and increasing movement are less consistent than the results of DBS on the globus pallidus or the subthalamic nucleus. Pallidotomy is done on the side of the brain opposite the side of the most dyskinesia or the most severe bradykinesia. Bilateral simultaneous pallidotomy carries the risk of speech and thinking difficulty. As with any surgery, there are risks, especially with older people. There is a 1% to 3% risk of stroke or hemorrhage with thalamotomy or pallidotomy.

70. What is DBS?

Stimulation surgery or **deep brain stimulation** (DBS) refers to implanting a probe or electrode, a stimulator into a clearly defined, abnormally discharging brain region—a region generating "static." This is usually, but not always, the same region targeted in ablative or destructive surgery. By generating a blocking or inhibiting counter-current, the effects of the static are lessened or negated. Technically, DBS is a misnomer—the abnormal discharging brain region isn't stimulated; rather, it's blocked or inhibited by a reverse or counter-current.

Deep brain stimulation

a treatment in which a probe or electrode is implanted and used to stimulate a clearly defined, abnormally discharging brain region to block the abnormal activity.

There is renewed interest in DBS because is it seen as a refinement of thalamotomy and pallidotomy. However, instead of destroying a section of brain tissue, DBS uses a high-frequency electrical charge to stimulate the brain. Where the electrode is placed in the brain determines which symptoms will be alleviated. Two surgeries are required. In one surgery, a microelectrode is implanted in a specific region to remain there permanently. Wires from the implanted electrode are then passed beneath the skin to a small battery pack placed under the skin near the shoulder. This device is then adjusted to the patient's own needs to regulate the frequency in the electrode. The patient will be able to turn it off and on by means of a magnet. When the device is on, the stimulation will stop the tremor, the dyskinesia, or improve bradykinesia within a few seconds. When it is turned off, the tremor or dyskinesia will return. The major advantage of this surgery is that it has fewer complications than thalamotomy or pallidotomy, and there is significant improvement of symptoms, sometimes requiring smaller amounts of PD drugs. The regions targeted by DBS are the thalamus, the globus pallidus, and the subthalamic nucleus. Increasingly, the subthalamic nucleus is becoming the preferred target. The subthalamic nucleus is located below the thalamus, and it acts as "brake" on the substantia nigra. Studies have compared DBS to thalamotomy and pallidotomy, and although sufficient data still need to be collected, these studies have shown promising results in favor of DBS.

71. What is restorative surgery?

Restorative or transplantation surgery transfers or implants dopamine-producing cells into the striatum. The striatum, from the Latin "stripped-substance," is named because of the large number of fibers that cross it—giving it a stripped or braided appearance. In the striatum fibers project downward from the cerebral cortex, co-mingling with dopamine fibers projecting upward from the substantia nigra. The striatum is composed of two parts: the caudate nucleus and the putamen. The putamen is more affected in PD.

Cells are transplanted into the striatum because it's easier and safer to locate and target than the smaller and less accessible substantia nigra. Because the foreign cells aren't transplanted into the nigra, they can't replicate exactly the lost nigral cells. As an example, dopamine cells in the nigra receive, exchange, analyze, process, and interpret information from other brain regions including serotonin cells in the brainstem (a region below the nigra) and the subthalamic nucleus. Dopamine cells transplanted into the striatum don't receive, exchange, analyze, process, and interpret information from the brain stem or subthalamic nucleus.

Transplanted cells can come from several sources. Once implanted, the cells then attempt to compensate for the lost cells in the patient's substantia nigra. There are 400,000 nerve cells in the substantia nigra, with 200,000 on each side. When a person loses 240,000 cells, 60% of his total, PD first appears. This implies that 160,000 cells, or 40%, are the minimum needed to maintain normal movement. Approximately 80–90% of transplanted cells die during implantation, failing to take hold or establish connections within the patient's brain. Successful transplantation usually requires at least 1.6 million cells, 10 times the minimum. If human embryos are used, transplantation requires at least 3 to 4 embryos with 400,000 cells in each embryo.

Transplantation or restorative surgery seeks to reestablish dopamine levels in the brain while setting back the "PD clock," returning the patient to a less advanced disease stage. Transplantation is usually performed bilaterally. In some hospitals surgery is performed on both sides at the same setting. In other hospitals surgery is performed in stages: first one side, then several weeks or months later, the other side. The surgery is performed stereotactically—that is, with the patient asleep. The surgery carries approximately the same risks as ablative surgery: a 1% to 3% risk of hemorrhage, stroke, or death. Unlike ablative surgery or DBS, the benefits of transplantation aren't apparent for months—because the transplanted cells must establish integrate themselves into the patient's brain.

Most, but not all, patients who undergo transplantation surgery are treated with immunosuppressive drugs to prevent the brain from rejecting the cells. There's a difference of opinion among researchers as to the necessity of using immunosuppressive drugs. Sources of transplanted cells include:

- *Cells from the patient's adrenal gland.* These cells resemble but are not identical to dopamine producing cells. This approach was successful in very few patients. Most PD patients had difficulty undergoing simultaneous operations: one on their belly to remove their adrenal gland, then one their brain to implant the adrenal gland. The survival of adrenal tissue in the brain is poor. This approach was abandoned.
- *Cells from the patient's carotid body.* A small cluster of dopamine-producing cells encircle the carotid artery in the neck. These cells are removed and implanted into the patient's brain. This operation has had limited success—probably because there aren't enough cells in the carotid body to implant into the brain.
- *Cells from aborted human embryos.* This approach, and much of our knowledge of human transplanta-

tion was pioneered by Bjorkland and Lindvall (Sweden). The social and ethical concerns surrounding the use of human embryos, the difficulty of obtaining an adequate number of embryos, and the dissimilarity among embryos has limited this surgery. Human embryos must be collected at 9 to 12 weeks gestation, as only such embryos contain cells that can differentiate into dopamine producing cells. The embryos and their donors are screened for viruses and other infectious agents to prevent spreading disease to the recipient. The embryonic tissue is usually transplanted into the putamen. The putamen, more than the caudate nucleus, is involved in directing and regulating movement. After several months, the transplanted tissue integrates itself into the brain and acts as a pump injecting dopamine directly into the putamen—where's it's deficient. A study conducted in a randomized, double-blind manner including "sham" surgery demonstrated transplantation is moderately beneficial in some patients—predominantly those less than 60 years.

- *Cells from pig embryos.* Pigs are immunologically close to humans. An unlimited number—millions and millions—of cells from specifically bred, developed, and prepared pig embryos can be made available for transplantation. The results with pig transplants have, however, been disappointing.
- *Spheramine.* Spheramine consists of normal human cells (pigmented cells from the human retina) that provide dopamine and that are attached to microcarriers. In a pilot study, millions of spheramine cells were delivered unilaterally to the brain with modest improvement.

72. *What are stem cells?*

Stem cells are primitive cells that have the ability to divide countless times and to give rise to specialized cells. Life begins when a sperm fertilizes an egg and creates a single cell that has the potential to be a human being. This fertilized egg is called totipotent because it can generate every cell in the body; this is an embryonic stem cell. In the first hours after fertilization, this cell divides into identical totipotent cells. If placed into a woman's uterus, either of these cells can develop into a human being. In fact, identical twins develop when two totipotent cells separate and develop into two genetically identical human beings.

Four days after fertilization and after several cycles of cell division, these totipotent cells specialize, forming a hollow sphere called a blastocyst. The cyst has an outer and an inner layer of cells. The outer cells will form the placenta; the inner cells will form all the tissues of the human body. Although the inner cells, known as pluripotent cells (or embryonic stem cells), form almost every type of human cell, they cannot form a human being. Because they are not totipotent, they are not embryos. If the inner cells were placed into a woman's uterus, they would not develop into a human being.

The pluripotent cells undergo specialization into stem cells that subsequently produce cells that have a particular function. Examples of these stem cells include blood stem cells, which give rise to red blood cells, white blood cells and platelets, and skin stem cells, which form the various types of skin tissue. These stem cells are called multipotent and are present in the bone marrow of all people.

A technique called somatic cell nuclear transfer (SCNT) isolates pluripotent stem cells. Using SCNT, researchers take a normal animal egg cell and remove the nucleus (the structure containing the chromosomes). The material left behind in the egg contains nutrients that are essential for embryo development. Any cell other than an egg or a sperm cell is then placed next to the egg from which the nucleus has been removed, and the two are fused. The resulting fused cell and its immediate descendants are totipotent; that is, they have the potential to develop into an entire animal. These totipotent cells will form a blastocyst. Cells from the inner cells of the blastocyst could, in theory, be used to develop pluripotent stem cell lines. At the most fundamental level, pluripotent stem cells can help us understand the events that occur during human development. A goal of this work is the identification of the process that results in cell specialization. We know that turning genes on and off is central to this process, but we do not know much about these "decision-making" genes or what turns them on or off. Some of our most serious medical conditions, such as cancer and birth defects, are due to abnormal cell specialization and cell division. A better understanding of normal cell processes may allow us to correct these conditions.

Human pluripotent stem cell research may dramatically change the way we develop drugs and test them for safety. For example, new drugs could be initially tested using human cell lines. Cell lines are currently used in this way (in cancer research, for example). Pluripotent stem cells would allow testing in more cell types, which would streamline the process of drug development. Only the drugs that are both safe and effective in cell line testing would graduate to further testing in laboratory animals and human subjects.

The most far-reaching potential of human pluripotent stem cells is the generation of cells and tissue that could be used in "cell therapies." Many diseases result from disruption of cellular function or destruction of tissues. Today, donated organs and tissues are often used to replace ailing organs. However, the number of people suffering from these disorders outpaces the number of organs available for transplantation. Pluripotent stem cells, stimulated to develop into specialized cells, offer the possibility of a renewable source of replacement cells and tissue to treat PD, Alzheimer disease, spinal cord injury, stroke, burns, heart disease, diabetes, and arthritis.

Adult Stem Cells. Multipotent stem cells can be found in some types of adult tissue, including that of the nervous system. In fact, stem cells are needed to replenish the cells in our body that wear out normally. In humans, neuronal stem cells have been isolated from fetal tissue and a cell that may be a neuronal stem cell has been isolated from adult brain tissue. Do adult stem cells have the same potential as pluripotent stem cells? Until recently, there was little evidence that multipotent cells such as blood stem cells could change course and produce skin cells, liver cells or any cell other than a blood cell. However, research is leading scientists to question this view. In animals, it has been shown that some adult stem cells previously thought to be committed to the development of one line of specialized cells are able to develop into other types of specialized cells. For example, recent experiments suggest that when neural stem cells are placed into the bone marrow, they produced a variety of blood cell types. Other studies have indicated that stem cells found in the bone marrow are able to produce liver cells. This suggests that even after a stem cell has begun to specialize, the stem cell may, under certain conditions, be more flexible.

Research suggests that these multipotent cells have great potential for use in both research and in the development of cell therapies. For example, there would be advantages to using adult stem cells for transplantation. If we could isolate the adult stem cells from a patient, coax them to divide and direct their specialization, and then transplant them back into the patient, these cells would *not* be rejected. The use of adult stem cells for such cell therapies would reduce or even avoid using stem cells that were derived from human embryos, sources that trouble many people on ethical grounds.

While adult stem cells hold promise, there are limitations to what we may or may not be able to accomplish with them. Thus, although many different kinds of multipotent stem cells have been identified, adult stem cells for all cell and tissue types have not yet been found in the adult human. Second, adult stem cells are often present in only small quantities, are difficult to isolate and purify, and their numbers may decrease with age. Any attempt to use stem cells from a patient's own body for treatment would require that stem cells first be isolated from the patient and then grown in culture in sufficient numbers to obtain adequate quantities for treatment. For some disorders, there may not be time to grow enough cells to use for treatment. In other disorders that are caused by a genetic defect, the genetic error would likely be present in the patient's stem cells. Cells from such a patient would not be appropriate for transplantation. There is evidence that stem cells from adults may not have the same capacity to grow as younger cells do. Moreover, adult stem cells may contain more DNA abnormalities, caused by exposure to daily living, including sunlight, toxins, and by the expected errors made in DNA replication during a person's lifetime. These weaknesses could limit the usefulness of adult stem cells. The development of stem cell lines, both pluripotent and multipotent, that may produce many human tissues, is an important scientific breakthrough. It is not too unrealistic to say that this research has the potential to revolutionize the practice of medicine and improve the quality and length of life.[1]

---

[1]The above was adapted by Dr. Lieberman from his National Institute of Health (NIH) article that appeared in May 2000.

PART SEVEN

Other Approaches to PD

Should I exercise?

What should I eat?

Why am I losing weight?

More...

73. Should I exercise?

Exercise will not stop or reverse the progression of PD, but it can improve your body strength and muscle tone so that you will be less disabled. Regular exercise is important to everyone, including people with PD. It can become one of your best strategies for coping with PD; besides the physical benefits, exercise can lift depression and improve your mood. Although even healthy people have difficulty sticking to an exercise program, it is even harder for someone with PD. Stiffness, fatigue, limited movements, and even difficulty breathing make exercise more challenging. If exercise used to be a joy and you were able to experience improvement in strength and endurance, with PD, it may not be so. Don't become discouraged, because although the gains may not be world class, you are strengthening your resistance and creating a better quality of life.

Exercise must be personalized. If you have been playing tennis, golfing, riding a bike, or jogging, continue to do it for as long as you can. Walking a mile or more every day is good exercise, and swimming is beneficial. However, if you have "off" periods, be certain there is someone around when you swim. Calisthenics done alone or with a partner every morning are good for both of you, and they can be tailored to match your physical capabilities. Keeping your muscles and joints active and flexible will keep them, and you, functioning longer. Make your exercise part of your daily routine.

Not all exercise is dull, repetitive, or tiring. Some activities of daily living are a form of exercise. Cleaning the house, working in the yard, doing chores, and going shopping are a type of exercise, too. They may not bulk up your muscles or improve your heart rate, but they will keep you flexible and limber. Try Tai Chi or yoga, which are very good for maintaining flexibility. Tailoring an exercise program to your particular needs may require working with a physical therapist trained in PD. Thus, if your problem is rigidity of the trunk, your exercise program may be different than if your problem is rigidity of your arms or legs. If your problem is curvature or flexion of your spine, you may require a different program than you would if your problem is flexion of your feet.

74. What should I eat?

Just as no food or diet is known to cause PD, neither of these is known to prevent or slow the progression of PD. The best diet you can eat is a balanced diet with plenty of fruits, vegetables, whole grains, and protein. Because processing of food in the digestive tract becomes slower for people with PD, eating lots of roughage becomes more important for maintaining good bowel habits and avoid constipation. Adding extra vegetables like carrots, broccoli, cauliflower, and cabbage along with extra fiber from cereals like bran can help. The addition of prunes or dried figs and apricots to the diet works for many people. Prunes now come flavored with orange or lemon, and a couple of prunes make a sweet and delicious treat. Drinking extra water, even if you don't feel thirsty, is also helpful. A glass of wine or beer or an alcoholic beverage can also be enjoyed in moderation. There is no need to eliminate any particular food or drink you enjoy—even chocolate is allowed!

One specific food that people with PD often ask questions about is fava beans. Fava beans contain levodopa, the precursor to dopamine, and were the original source of levodopa. However, depending on where they were grown and which part of the plant is used, the amount of levodopa present can vary considerably. It has been estimated that 3 ounces of fava beans contain about 250 mg of levodopa, but without carbidopa, the enzyme that metabolizes levodopa, to break it down, barely 50 mg of levodopa is available. Fava beans are an excellent source of both vitamins and roughage in the diet, but there is no reason to favor them over any other. Fava beans have been and are being eaten as a source of levodopa. In a small number of people who lack a specific enzyme called glucose–6-phosphate dehydrogenase (G6PD), there is a risk of a condition called hemolytic anemia. The enzyme can be identified by a blood test. If there is a question as to whether you have this condition, discuss eating fava beans with your doctor.

75. Why am I losing weight?

About 10% of people with PD lose weight. This usually happens late in PD, but weight loss may occur early. Weight loss occurs with decreased food intake, increased metabolism, or both. In PD, weight loss may occur for the following reasons:

- Decreased appetite may be caused by anxiety or depression, or by drugs such as Sinemet (which may also cause nausea). A decreased sense of smell (part of PD) often results in decreased sense of taste and less desire for food.

- Difficulty eating can cause you to eat more slowly and become satiated more easily; thus, you eat less.
- Decreased ability to swallow can also cause you to become satiated more easily, so you eat less.
- Increased physical activity. Patients who have frequent, moderate to marked tremors, dyskinesia, or rigidity burn calories faster.

Eating involves using your hands to hold a fork, knife, and spoon, carrying the food from your plate to your mouth, holding the food in your mouth, chewing, and then swallowing it. PD may affect your ability to perform any or all of these steps. Although each of these tasks may be affected minimally, cumulatively, the affect on eating can be marked. As an example, try chewing food while doing the following: (1) not moving your cheeks, (2) not moving your lips, and (3) not moving your tongue. Each movement is affected in PD, so the effect on eating can be marked. Although unaware, some people with PD flex their heads and touch their chin to their chest. This makes chewing and swallowing difficult. Try chewing and swallowing a mouthful of food with your chin touching your chest. It's not easy because this position does not allow your muscles of mastication (the muscles used for chewing) to operate at a mechanical advantage, and your throat isn't in a straight line with your esophagus. Now try chewing and swallowing with your head up. It's easy because this position allows your muscles of mastication to operate at a mechanical advantage and your throat is in a straight line with your esophagus. If you're having difficulty eating and the difficulty is out of proportion to your other symptoms, try to do the following:

- Take a dose of Sinemet an hour before you eat, on an empty stomach. This results in Sinemet's maximum absorption. Then when you're ready to eat, all of your muscles—in your hands, cheeks, tongue, and lips—are ready.
- Sit with your elbows on the table. This is not what your mother taught you, but she didn't know about PD. Sitting with your elbows on the table forces you, without your realizing it, to hold your head up. This will help you to better chew and swallow your food.

It's thought but not proven that in PD the hypothalamus (a region in the brain that controls all the glands and the ANS) is reset and causes the body to burn calories more quickly. If you're losing weight, eating well, and don't have a marked tremor or dyskinesia, causes of weight loss other than PD must be considered. These include cancer; depression; diabetes; drugs, such as high doses of Sinemet, amphetamines, cancer chemotherapy drugs, cocaine, laxatives, lithium, or thyroid drugs; diseases of the stomach (ulcers) or intestines (colitis, diverticulitis); infections, including AIDS and tuberculosis; and thyroid disease, or overactivity.

A useful rule in PD is to weigh yourself regularly and to keep a record of your weight. Then, if you see a downward trend, you may be able to relate it to a particular event: when you started a certain drug, when you began to have trouble swallowing. See your doctor when weight loss is excessive. The doctor may ask you the following:

When did the weight loss begin? Has it been sudden or gradual? How much have you lost? Has your appetite decreased? Has the amount or kinds of food you eat changed? Has your physical activity increased? Have you been sick? Have you had problems with your teeth or gums? Has your mouth been sore? Have you been anxious or depressed? Have you been nauseated? Have you been vomiting? Have you been more fatigued or tired? Have you had diarrhea? Have you been constipated? Have you had episodes when your heart pounds, you sweat, and you feel hungry (suggesting hypoglycemia)? Have you been excessively thirsty (suggesting diabetes)? Have you been urinating excessively (also indicating diabetes)? Has your hair been thinning or falling out (possibly due to thyroid disease)? What drugs—including alcohol, diuretics, laxatives, lithium, and PD drugs—are you taking.?

The doctor will then do a physical examination including a measurement of your weight. How extensive and detailed the evaluation for weight loss will depend upon information the doctor has gathered from the questions above. Once the cause is found, a consultation with a registered dietitian is a must.

76. Should I avoid protein?

Early in PD, wearing off and on-off do not occur and people on a three-times-per-day dose of Sinemet do not have to worry about restricting protein. As PD advances, as people on Sinemet develop wearing off and on-off, paying attention to protein can make a difference. This is because dietary protein causes a large peak in the concentration of certain amino acids that circulate in the bloodstream an hour after meals. These amino acids share with levodopa a "carrier" that transports them across the gut wall into the bloodstream and another "carrier" that transports them across the blood brain barrier. When blood amino acid levels are high, levodopa uptake into the brain is low. When this happens, people "turn off" and their PD symptoms reappear. Additional studies in PD indicate that anything that slows the speed of gastric emptying will slow the entry of levodopa into the blood and into the brain. Some of the drugs used to treat PD slow gastric emptying, including Artane and Cogentin. However, the chief culprit is food. For this reason it's best to take Sinemet on an empty stomach. Although levodopa absorption from the stomach into the bloodstream and from the bloodstream into the brain would be optimal if people ate no protein, without protein it would not be possible to maintain good nutrition. Protein provides one of the main components of our diet, along with carbohydrates and fats. It's possible, however, to modify your diet in such a way that all of your body's requirement for protein, at least 40 grams a day, can be eaten in a single evening meal.

When people find that a protein redistribution diet does not help with their wearing off or on-off, it is usually because they are unaware of the protein content of their food. The foods that contain little or no protein are, for the most part, vegetables and fruits. These can be eaten fresh, frozen, canned, stewed, or dried states and their juices can be consumed as well.

High protein foods are meat, poultry, fish, eggs, all dairy products (except butter), beans, and nuts. Cake made with milk and eggs is a high protein food. Pasta and bread contain a great deal of protein, but low protein forms of each can be found. If you are eating a protein-limited diet, you must be careful that you are getting enough calories from the other foods that you are eating. Together with swallowing difficulties and other problems, eating can become so troublesome that weight loss and malnutrition can result. The help of a dietician can make a difficult diet more palatable and nutritional.[2]

77. Do I need vitamins?

Health foods, nutritional supplements, and high doses of vitamins have *not* been shown in scientifically conducted studies, as opposed to anecdotal stories and paid testimonials, to help in PD. People with PD have the same requirements for vitamins as anyone, and if you eat a balanced diet, you will get all of the vitamins that you need. Two vitamins are of special interest in PD.

Pyridoxine, or vitamin B6, was thought to help PD when it was discovered in 1938. In 1950, however, the American Medical Association concluded that vitamin B6 did not help PD. Then B6 was found to be a cofactor, or **coenzyme**, for **dopa decarboxylase**, the enzyme that changes levodopa to dopamine. Based on this observation, B6 in doses 1,000 times higher than necessary for nutrition was given, without effect, to people

Coenzyme
molecules that enable enzymes to act more efficiently.

Dopa decarboxylase
the enzyme that changes levodopa to dopamine.

---

[2]Adapted with permission from *Parkinson's Disease: Guidelines for Medical Nutrition Therapy* by Kathrynne Holden, MS, RD. For more information on nutrition and PD, call 877–565–2665 or visit *www.nutritionucanlivewith.com.*

with PD. Again, interest in B6 faded. After levodopa, without carbidopa, was introduced as a treatment for PD, it was found that B6, in small doses (15 mg per day), blocked the effects of levodopa. This sparked an interest in multivitamin preparations lacking B6 and caused people with PD to avoid B6. When carbidopa was combined with levodopa in Sinemet, it was found that small doses of B6 no longer blocked levodopa. If you are on Sinemet or Madopar (the European equivalent of Sinemet), it takes at least 50 mg of B6, more than is available in most multivitamin preparations, to block Sinemet or Madopar. Vitamin B6, in non-blocking doses, occurs naturally in tomatoes, soybeans, bran, and brewers' yeast.

Tocopherol, or *Vitamin E,* is an antioxidant that helps prevent damage from free radicals. Free radicals arise from the breakdown and oxidation of foods and naturally occurring body chemicals. Damage from free radicals may be implicated in the death of the dopamine cells in PD. At one time, doctors thought that high doses of vitamin E (2,000 units per day) might slow the progression of PD. However, a large National Institutes of Health study (called DATATOP) found no evidence that vitamin E slowed the progression of PD. Despite this study, claims continue to be made that vitamin E slows the progression of PD. The claims are based on a theory that differences between naturally occurring and synthetic forms of vitamin E could explain why DATATOP showed no benefit for vitamin E. Although the natural form of vitamin E is two to three times as potent as the synthetic form, contains all the tocopherols (all the different forms of vitamin E), and is better absorbed, there's no scientific basis for the claim. There's a role for vitamin E in nutrition, and its merits should be discussed with a dietitian; however, there's no evidence of a special role for vitamin E in PD. The best source of vitamin E is from foods that contain all of the various tocopherols (forms) of vitamin E. Good food sources of vitamin E are nuts and seeds, avocados, mayonnaise, wheat germ, peanut butter, dark green leafy vegetables, and asparagus. The recommendation for vitamin E is 22 units a day with a safe limit of up to 1,000 units a day. Remember, you can buy a drug or a vitamin without a doctor's prescription, but this does not mean that it is safe. Thus, if you're taking "blood thinners" such as aspirin, warfarin (coumadin), or clopidogrel (Plavix) you should ask your doctor whether it safe to use vitamin E. Large amounts of vitamin E (100 to 200 units per day) can interfere with these drugs and result in your blood clotting more easily.[3]

78. What is Coenzyme Q–10?

Although considered a vitamin, Coenzyme Q–10 (CoQ10 for short), which is chemically related to vitamin K, is not a vitamin. Vitamins are substances not made in the body; CoQ10 is made in the body, but perhaps not in sufficient quantities. CoQ10 is an "over-the-counter" preparation, which means you do not need a doctor's prescription to buy it. As you age you make less CoQ10, and it's possible that a deficiency can develop. In addition, some conditions, including heart failure, renal failure, and, perhaps PD, can use up your

---

[3]Adapted with permission from *Parkinson's Disease: Guidelines for Medical Nutrition Therapy* by Kathrynne Holden, MS, RD. For more information on nutrition and PD, call 877–565–2665 or visit *www.nutritionucanlivewith.com.*

Statins

supplements used to
lower cholesterol
that may also slow
the progression of
PD.

body's store of CoQ10. In addition, some drugs can interfere with the action of CoQ10 or decrease its production. Such drugs include the **statins**, widely used to lower cholesterol. Indeed, some doctors routinely prescribe CoQ10 supplements for their patients who are taking statins such as Leschol, Lipitor, Mevacor, Pravachol, or Zocor. These drugs may also include certain diabetic drugs, including beta-blockers such as propranolol and metoprolol, and certain common tranquillizers such as Compazine, Stellazine, and Thorazine.

CoQ10 MAY slow the rate of progression of PD. CoQ10 may do so in two ways: (1) CoQ10 is an antioxidant, and this property may have a role in slowing the rate of progression of PD. (2) However, the main role of CoQ10 in slowing the rate of progression of PD may be its property as an energy source. Muscle, brain, liver, and platelets are rich in CoQ10. Each of your body's 100 trillion cells has its own energy source, a series of "battery packs" called **mitochondria**. These structures allow each cell, including the brain's dopamine cells, to do what they're supposed to do. CoQ10 is important in the operation of the "battery packs": CoQ10 transfers energy from a battery, called Complex I, to another battery called Complex II. In PD, there is a deficiency of Complex I in *platelets* (a blood component). It's not known whether there's a similar deficiency in the brain's dopamine-producing cells. A deficiency of CoQ10 may be responsible for the deficiency of Complex I, hence the interest in CoQ10 in PD. A recent study in a small number of people with PD suggests that CoQ10 in high doses (1,200 mg per day) may slow the rate of progression of PD. Until this study, the highest amounts of CoQ10 used were 400 mg per day. Although the study is

Mitochondria

cellular energy
sources.

promising, it has also raised questions about the safety of high doses of CoQ10. This is an issue that should be discussed with your doctor.

CoQ10 is present in small amounts in certain foods, including meats, liver, unsaturated oils, and nuts. The recommended dose of CoQ10 based on past studies is 30 to 300 mg daily. These recommendations may increase. It's best to take CoQ10 in divided doses, twice a day rather than all at once, to aid absorption. CoQ10 is fat soluble, and the oil-based soft gel is better absorbed than dry tablets or capsules. Because it can auto-oxidize, it is best taken with 100 units of vitamin E. CoQ10 and vitamin E may work synergistically (better together than separately).

79. Is NutraSweet bad for PD?

Aspartame (NutraSweet) is composed of two amino acids, aspartic acid and the methyl ester of phenylalanine. When aspartame is absorbed, about 10% of the dose is converted to methanol, which is then converted to formaldehyde, then to carbon dioxide and water. All of these conversions occur by normal metabolic processes. These same processes are used in converting the methanol found in many fruits, fruit juices, vegetables, and wine to carbon dioxide and water. Thus, methanol is a natural by-product of the metabolism of many commonly eaten foods. In fact, a glass of tomato juice provides about 5 times as much methanol as a similar amount of diet soft drink containing aspartame. These amounts of methanol from many foods, or the lesser amounts from aspartame, are rapidly metabolized, do not accumulate in the body, and do not reach harmful amounts.

The small amounts of methanol formed by the metabolism of aspartame (comparable to that occurring in fruit juices) have been alleged, in uncontrolled studies, to be a factor in diseases such as PD. The presence of phenylalanine in aspartame has been alleged, in uncontrolled studies, to block the absorption of levodopa, and to aggravate PD. PD existed before aspartame was invented, and there is no evidence, however, that aspartame causes or aggravates PD.

The safety of aspartame has been established, and consumption of diet soft drinks or other foods containing aspartame is not associated with adverse health effects. The level of daily consumption that is judged to be safe by the FDA is 50 milligrams per kilogram (mg/kg) of body weight per day. At this level, for example, a 150-pound (60-kilogram) person would need to consume almost 16 12-ounce cans of a beverage containing aspartame to reach this level of intake.

80. Is coffee good for PD?

There have been studies that suggest that caffeine protects against PD. Thus, if your drink several cups of coffee a day, and have been doing so for many years, you may be 30% less likely to have PD. However, care must be taken in how these data are interpreted. Although it was found that people who drank coffee or other caffeine containing beverages such as tea, cocoa, and cola had lower incidences of PD, other explanations are possible. It could be that as PD develops, with its tremors and sleep problems, people with PD begin to avoid caffeine. Another explanation might be that people with a tendency to develop PD have a physiological or psychological intolerance to caffeine.

In one study, men who drank large quantities of coffee or other caffeinated beverages had a lower risk of PD than men who drank only a little. The study suggested that it is the caffeine consumed before the onset of PD that provides the protection, whereas caffeine consumed after PD develops provides none. In women, the protective effects of caffeine are harder to evaluate. In moderate amounts, caffeine appears to offer some protection from PD in women. However, at increased levels of consumption, the benefit is lost, and a reverse effect is observed. This may have a biological explanation, or perhaps women have a different susceptibility to PD. Obviously more studies are needed.

If you enjoy drinking coffee, continue to do so. If you don't, don't start drinking it because it might prevent PD. And if you have PD, drinking or not drinking coffee will not make a difference. Starbucks is a wonderful place, but it's not the answer to PD.

81. Is smoking good for PD?

Several studies suggest cigarette smoking may protect against developing PD. Thus, if you smoke one or two packs a day and have been doing so for many years, you may be about 50% less likely to have PD. These studies indicate that the degree of protection is related to the number of packs smoked per day, and the number of years of smoking. There is no evidence, however, that once PD begins, smoking is protective. At different times it has been proposed that certain chemicals in cigarette smoke, not yet identified, may have a protective effect. Some researchers, noting the loss of smell in people with PD, have proposed that PD may result from an "inhaled" agent, and smoking may block this agent. Some researchers have observed that nicotine, by stimulating nicotine receptors in the brain, may relieve somewhat some of the symptoms of PD. Other researchers are skeptical. They point out that cigarette smoking, by decreasing life span, may "kill off" those people who would have developed PD. Other researchers point out that PD is a slowly evolving disease that begins years before it is diagnosed. These researchers think that an early loss of desire to smoke may, actually, be an early symptom of PD. Instead of viewing smoking as neuro-protective, they believe that people who do not take up smoking or stop smoking may already have PD.

To test the idea that cigarette smoking may protect against the development of PD, in 1999 a study was conducted by Drs. Carly Tanner and J. William Langston of the California Parkinson Institute. The study is summarized below:

> Smoking has been inversely associated with PD, but whether this reflects a biologic effect on the underlying disease process or merely selection bias is uncertain. The authors compared smoking histories in male twin pairs identified from the National Academy of Sciences–National Research Council World War II Veteran Twins. The amount of cigarettes smoked (in pack-years) was collected until the time of PD onset in the affected twin or until the time of death for the unaffected twin. Differences in pack-years smoked until PD onset and until 10 and 20 years before onset were compared using standard statistical methods. To assess the role of shared environment, correlation for smoking behaviors was compared between pairs, both of whom had PD and pairs where only one of the

twins had PD. Detailed smoking histories were available for 113 twin pairs.

There were 43 identical twins and 50 non identical twins in which at least one twin had .

There were 10 identical twins and 10 non-identical twins in which both twins had PD. In 33 identical twins and 39 non-identical twins in which at least one twin had PD and smoked, the twins without PD smoked more than the twins with PD. This was more marked in the identical twins than in the non-identical twins. In twins the risk of PD is inversely correlated with the dose (in pack-years) of cigarette smoking: the less you smoke the more likely you are to develop PD. Because identical twins are genetically identical and are similar behaviorally, this difference is unlikely to result from either genetic or other environmental factors. These results are compatible with a true protective effect of cigarette smoking.

Although studies suggest smoking may be protective against PD, the risks of smoking in causing cancer, heart disease, and stroke, far outweigh any potential benefit in preventing PD: if you don't smoke, don't start because of PD. More needs to be understood about how smoking protects against PD before recommendations can be made.

82. Is hormone replacement therapy (HRT) good for PD?

Estrogen replacement can relieve hot flashes, which in some people can be debilitating. This is of concern to women with PD, whose risk for osteoporosis is increased. Also, although studies are not conclusive, there is evidence that estrogen may protect against PD. Evidence for this is small but tantalizing. More men than women have PD: 55 men for every 45 women. Estrogen may modulate dopamine receptors. Some premenopausal women report that their PD drugs are ineffective during ovulation (the middle of the menstrual cycle) and shortly before the start of their monthly menses, when estrogen levels are low.

At menopause, women stop making estrogen, and for years have been prescribed an estrogen made from the urine of pregnant horses (Premarin) and progestin, a synthetic form of the hormone progesterone (Provera). The combination is called Prempro. The treatment was originally given to relieve such symptoms as hot flashes, but later to reduce bone thinning and heart disease. Estrogen alone relieved symptoms but produced a small increase in the risk for cancer of the uterus), so the synthetic progestin was added to lower this risk. But did estrogen or an estrogen–progestin combination really reduce the risk of heart disease? Two studies cast doubt on the safety of both estrogen and estrogen–progestin therapies. However, many doctors do not think the results of these studies are a reason to stop HRT.

To judge whether you are a candidate for HRT remember: (1) HRT will not prevent heart disease and may increase it. (2) HRT will help to prevent bone thinning, and this is a consideration for women with a family history of osteoporosis. However, there are natural forms of estrogen along with supplements of minerals and vitamins, as well as weight-bearing exercise, also help to prevent bone thinning. (3) HRT slightly decreases risk for colorectal cancer, an important consideration for those who have PD, or those with a family history of colorectal cancer, but it also may increase the risk of breast cancer. (4) If you do not have hot flashes, or if they are mild, you don't require medication. (4) Nutrition and exercise may be a much higher priority than HRT. If you, like some women, find that your PD symptoms are decreased with HRT, then that could be a good reason to continue the therapy, if your doctor agrees.

At this time, the best advice is to take the lowest possible amount of hormones that is effective for you. Your doctor can measure hormone levels in your blood or saliva to determine the correct amount for you. You may want to consider using natural hormones, also known as "bio-identical hormones." One source for bio-identical hormones is the Women's International Pharmacy, whose pharmacists will work together with your doctor to compound a preparation for you.[4]

83. Should I take glutathione?

Glutathione is known to be an important antioxidant in the body and the brain. Glutathione is a tri-peptide, that is, it is made up of three amino acids strung together. Glutathione and the enzymes related to its metabolism have been reported to be depleted in the substantia nigra of people with PD. Whether this precedes the loss of the dopamine cells, or is a consequence of their loss (fewer cells means less

---

[4]Adapted with permission from *Parkinson's Disease: Guidelines for Medical Nutrition Therapy* by Kathrynne Holden, MS, RD. For more information on nutrition and PD, call 877–565–2665 or visit *www.parkinson.org/askdiet.htm*

glutathione) is not known. The primary role of glutathione is to protect cells from free radicals, destructive chemicals formed during the course of normal metabolism and/or by exposure to various environmental toxins. Glutathione also enhances the function of other anti-oxidant compounds by keeping them in a form suitable for inactivation of free radicals.

In 1996 Italian researchers reported that in people with PD, intravenous glutathione, given twice a day for one month, resulted in a decrease in their disability. After glutathione administration was stopped, the beneficial effect would last for as long as 2 to 4 months. The study has never been repeated or performed in a way that would live up to the gold standard of **clinical trials**—the double-blind, placebo-controlled trial. Such a test of the effectiveness has only recently been started. Presently glutathione is being administered based on belief that it works, rather than on the basis of objective evidence. Many PD patients throughout the United States are taking glutathione, and many swear by it, though many do not. The alleged effectiveness of glutathione is likely more "Madison Avenue hype" than science.

Glutathione can be purchased without a doctor's prescription. The glutathione is dissolved in a solution and a qualified healthcare practitioner administers it directly into an arm vein. The solution is infused over a 15–20 min interval. The usual dose is 1400 mg of glutathione three times a week. Although there are videotapes that attest to the miraculous benefits of glutathione, knowledgeable doctors and skeptical patients are aware that videotapes do not tell the whole truth. It is surprising that the antioxidant glutathione

Clinical trials
carefully monitored scientific studies of new drugs or treatments using human subjects.

would decrease symptoms of PD, since its mechanism of action is to protect the internal environment against oxidative stress, not to release dopamine. There is, of course, the possibility that glutathione has other poorly understood effects that enhance the action of levodopa or endogenous dopamine. This however remains to be proven. It is also possible that the immediate and short-term benefits of glutathione are the result of a placebo effect. It is well known that treatments with substances that have no biological effects can lead to dramatic improvement in disease symptoms—often for many months—if the person believes he or she is receiving an active agent. A good reason for being skeptical about its claimed effects is that it is not known if glutathione even gets into the brain (if it crosses the blood brain barrier) and if it does, whether it gets into the cells of the substantia nigra. In summary, glutathione is an important antioxidant that may or may not eventually be proven to be useful for the treatment of PD.[5]

---

[5]The above was adapted from an article in *Parkinson's Disease Update*, a newsletter devoted to the most current medical, social and psychological aspects of PD. You can subscribe by calling 215–947–6648.

PART EIGHT

Making the Most of Life with PD

How do I meet other people with PD?

Why me? What did I do to deserve PD?

How can I make my home safe?

More ...

84. How do I meet other people with PD?

You are not alone! PD has a large and extensive support network. Several large national organizations, such as The National Parkinson Foundation, the Parkinson Disease Foundation (now merged into The Parkinson Foundation) and the American Parkinson Disease Association, that sponsor support groups throughout the country for PD patients and their families. Many hospitals and regional health centers also have support groups, and many patients have started groups of their own. A support group can be an important asset to your survival—a lot can happen when a group of determined people rally around one uniting cause! In addition to sharing their experiences with you, members of support groups can often teach you about services available in the community and other local resources. People in support groups stay well informed on the newest and best types of treatments or know when and where a new trial or study on PD is taking place. Support groups work to educate the community or promote public policy that benefits people with PD. Support groups may not be for everybody, but there are many different kinds of support groups, including some for young-onset PD and some for caregivers, so there might be one that is particularly useful for you.

If a support group is not for you, there are numerous Internet-based PD groups that can be accessed at your convenience. Given the nature of the Internet, however, caution is always wise. A wealth of information is available on the Internet, but always consider carefully the source and accuracy of the information. If it sounds too good to be true, it probably is; buyer, beware! is a good rule of thumb. The large national PD organizations listed above have Web pages that offer referrals and information that are soundly based and well researched, so check them out. Some organizations offer subscriptions to newsletters with current information about PD, such as the National Parkinson Foundation's *PD Update*, The Parkinson Disease Foundation's *PDF News*, and the American Parkinson Disease Association's *APDA Newsletter*.

85. Why me? What did I do to deserve PD?

First you might feel angry with God, and then you may feel angry with yourself for being angry with God. It might feel as though all of your faith in a Higher Power must surely have been a mistake. There are no good explanations for why this seeming unfairness descended on your life, and then, just when you think that you have it figured out, the pain and worry of PD are reinforced. Still, many people find their strength in spirituality. In their despair, they turn to God and find help through their faith. Their faith grows, although their body fails; nevertheless, they find tranquility and the strength to accept the things that they cannot explain. Do not neglect your spiritual nature. Seek the wisdom of your sacred texts; speak to the holy, wherever you find it, as it may be your best weapon as you fight against your disease. Find pleasure in small wonders: a flower, a pet, a child's laughter—even the sunshine after the rain.

If your belief in God is shaken, or even if you weren't sure you believed in God to begin with, you may take comfort in the verses of Isaiah. Isaiah, a Biblical prophet lived in dark and troubled times—much like you. The golden age of King David and Solomon had passed. The Kingdom of Israel split into two parts, and each part was threatened by enemies. Although Isaiah lived in troubled times and foresaw terrible events, he continued to believe. His poetry translated from Aramaic to Greek to Latin to English is as beautiful as any written. Although Isaiah's verses may have changed with each translation, his rhythms and themes are immortal.

Faith strengthens the weakened hands
The wilderness and the lonely place shall be glad for
* those who believe,*
And the desert shall rejoice and bloom as a rose.
And they who believe shall see the glory of God,
And the greatness of His works.
He will strengthen the weakened hands, and stifle the
* trembling knees.*

86. How can I make my home safe?

Look at the areas where you do most of your walking: from your bed to your bathroom, down the hall, to the kitchen, to the front or back door, and to your favorite chair in the living room. Make sure that those areas are safe for walking. Remove loose throw rugs, add extra lighting, and put night-lights where they will be the most helpful. Have rails installed along long stretches of hallway. Using motion detection devices on lamps in sitting areas will ensure light to see by and will reduce the hassle of turning it on manually. Move any obstacles out of the way to reduce chances of tripping and falling. Buy a long-handled mechanical tool for picking up things that drop to prevent unnecessary bending. A cordless phone that can be carried in a pocket or in the basket of a walker is a boon for catching calls without running to the phone. A television remote control with large buttons is another "user-friendly" device. If you have stairways in your home, make sure that the carpet isn't loose or that the steps aren't cracked. Putting reflective tape along the edges makes the steps more visible, especially at night. Make sure that the handrails are firmly attached and sturdy. Adding a second handrail on the other side may also prove useful. If doorknobs become troublesome, change them for lever-type door handles. Keys can be more easily managed if they are kept in a plastic holder that provides a grip as well as storage. Be sure to have good lighting at entryways—motion detectors or timers are useful here, too.

Most accidents in the house occur in the bathroom. Slipping and falling are the most prevalent here, so prevention is the goal. Small throw rugs on the floor can slip and slide or bunch up and cause falls. They should be removed and replaced with larger rugs that have non-slip backings. Adding grab bars to tub and shower walls helps to prevent falls, and grab bars near the toilet will help with getting up and down. An elevated toilet seat may also help with moving your bowels as well as make it easier for you to get on and off the seat. Be sure to put a rubber bath mat in the tub or shower to prevent slipping on the wet surface. Adding a bath stool or chair with rubber suction tips makes bathing easier, too. Buy soap on a rope or use shower gel from a tube to prevent slippery bars of soap from getting away. If faucet handles in the sink or shower are difficult to grasp, replace them with larger lever types. Handheld showerheads on long hoses are convenient and easy to use and can help you ensure that the water temperature is correct before you get in. Make sure that there are no glass containers in the bathroom; shampoo, hand cream, and mouthwash should all be purchased in plastic tubes or bottles. Exchange glass tumblers for paper cups to minimize the chances of breaking. Toothbrushes with fat handles make oral hygiene easier to manage, and electric shavers reduce the risk of nicks and cuts. In the bathroom, a nightlight is essential, and a large bell on the countertop or toilet tank makes it easy to summon help if needed.

Bedrooms should be comfortable, private areas that invite rest and relaxation. Be sure to have clear access to the bed, free of shoes or other clutter, and that the path to the bathroom is open. Because PD makes turning in bed slow and difficult, a blanket support at the foot of the bed allows feet to move freely. Satin sheets allow you to turn more easily. A firm mattress provides you with the support and leverage you need to turn more easily. If you're still having difficulty turning in bed it is probably because you do not raise your arm high enough to "flip you around in bed." Ask your partner to watch you turn in bed: if you're not raising your arm high enough you're not going to turn easily. Slippers should be easy to slip on your feet but not off, and they should have non-slip soles. A box of tissues, an accessible flashlight, and an unbreakable container of water on the nightstand will also come in handy. A nightlight with a motion detector that can switch on with the least movement can be useful. For men, a urinal can reduce trips to the bathroom. If a commode is necessary, be sure that it is placed as close to the bed as possible, with toilet tissue within easy reach. A plastic cloth on the floor beneath the commode can prevent spoiling the carpet in case of accidents or spills. A chair for dressing is indispensable, and it should have arms for ease in getting in and out. Other dressing aids include a long-handled shoehorn, a buttonhook, and a zipper pull.

87. What can I wear?

Perhaps one of the biggest problems could be shopping for clothes! Navigating through crowded malls, trying on clothes in small fitting rooms, and waiting on line to pay for your purchases takes the fun out of shopping and leaves a person with PD frustrated and exhausted. Instead, turn to mail-order catalogs and shop for clothing at home. Several companies carry items of clothing that are designed to be easier to put on and take off and still look very attractive. Men can wear pull on shirts, like the 3 button knit sport shirts, or in cold weather, they can wear turtlenecks: turtlenecks look great and are easy to wear. If dress shirts are necessary, try short-sleeve shirts: few people notice the absence of buttons or cufflinks. Clip-on ties can substitute for regular ties, which require you to tie a knot. And many clip-ins are indistinguishable from regular ties. For sportier or casual clothes, there are good looking pull-on pants with elastic waists that eliminate bothering with buttons or zippers. Shoes that close with Velcro are easier to wear than shoes that close with laces. And Velcro, unlike laces, does not break.

Slip-on loafers are an equally good choice. Some people with PD need rubber soles to grip the floor. Some people, especially those who freeze, need leather soles, soles that don't stick on carpets or catch on uneven surfaces and cause them to fall. Whether you need rubber or leather soles is determined by trial and error. You must try both and see which is best.

Women can wear skirts and slacks with elastic waists. They can also wear knit shirts, loose blouses, or pull-on sweaters. Bras that fasten in the front are simpler to put on. Bathrobes should be, at most, ankle length: floor length robes cause falls. Shoes should have flat or low heels and be easy to put on or take off.

88. How will I eat?

There are gadgets that help open jars of many different sizes, from catsup bottles to large mason jars. Electric canopeners are a boon, but you should find the one that is easy to use and hard to break. Electric knives may also seem like a good idea, but they're not, because if you slip, the cut is likely to be bigger and bloodier. Cutting boards that have suction feet can prevent slipping while cutting, and knives with larger handles are easier to use. If handles are not big enough for you to grip comfortably, they can be built up by taping on several layers of foam rubber until they fit your hand. Plastic handles that fit over half-gallon containers of juice or milk make the cartons easier to use. Cooking food in a crockpot allows different combinations of meat and vegetables to be cooked at the same time, producing tender, flavorful meals with a minimum of effort and reducing the possibility of burning either the food or the cook! Microwave ovens have simplified cooking for everyone, but be sure that the oven is easily accessible to minimize spilling hot liquids or foods. An electric broom makes cleaning up the floor a breeze, and the new soft cloth sweeping systems are better than a broom and dustpan.

Meal times for people with PD can be frustrating. Take the time you need to eat, don't hurry: hurrying can result in choking! Chew your food thoroughly before trying to swallow. If you're having trouble chewing lift up your chin. People with PD have a tendency to bend their neck (without realizing it) this results in your chin touching your chest. Try to chew with your chin touching your chest—it's hard. Now chew with your chin up—it's easier. You're using the same muscles but with your chin up you're using them at a mechanical advantage. If you can't remember to chew with your chin up, try keeping your elbows on the table. This is not what your mother taught you, but keeping your elbows on the table automatically forces your chin up. In some people eating smaller meals more frequently is helpful. If soup is on the menu, use a large-handled mug and drink it. Spoons may be more effective than forks for picking up food on your plate, and if your spoon has a large handle, it will be easier to use. Ask to have your meat cut into bite-size pieces in the kitchen so you don't have to struggle to cut it at table. Drinking straws work well when tremor makes drinking difficult. Never fill a cup or glass more than three quarters full: it's less likely to spill. A large bore straw rather than a narrow one is better. A damp washcloth makes a great napkin, especially when finger foods are served. A dining chair with arms makes it easier for the person with PD to steady their elbows and arms while eating. A strategically placed towel can protect your clothes from an accidental spill.

89. Will I be able to walk?

Staying mobile, and especially walking, is very important, so if you're having trouble and find yourself falling frequently, don't let pride keep you from enjoying life. People with PD develop difficulty walking, and some develop difficulty with balance; the two go together, but aren't the same because they result from different problems in the brain. Difficulty walking results in a shortened stride. Your steps become smaller, shorter and closer together, just as your handwriting may become smaller and more cramped, with letters and words closing together. Small, short steps can be helped sometimes by training, sometimes by a cane, sometimes by a walker. Difficulty with balance may also be helped through training (different from that for walking), sometimes by a cane, almost always by a walker.

The Curved Spine. If you walk with short steps: stand sideways and look in your mirror. Is your neck flexed on your chin? Are your shoulders rounded? Do they slope forward? Is your spine bent or curved? If the answer to two or three of the above is "yes," then the bent or curved spine may be part of the problem. The cause of the bent or curved or twisted spine is unknown. In some patients this results from an unequal pull of muscles in the front over muscles in the back of the spine. The spine is a fulcrum around which your hip, thigh, and back muscles exert leverage. If your spine is bent, curved, or twisted, or if your posture is stooped, you will not generate as much force with your hip, thigh, and back muscles. Consequently you take shorter, smaller steps than usual to cover a set distance and you fatigue easily. If your spine is straight, you generate more force with your hip, thigh, and back muscles, you take longer steps, you take fewer steps to cover a set distance, you walk more efficiently and you fatigue less.

To demonstrate how this works, try the following brief experiment:

1. Stand up and bend at your waist as far as you can.
2. Walk with your face down, your eyes looking at the floor, your spine curved like a letter "C."
3. Notice how you are forced to take small, short steps.

Keeping your spine straight, preventing your posture from becoming stooped is an important exercise. Here are some tips and an exercise that must be worked on all the time to keep your spine straight or to minimize the curve:

1. Learn to stand with your hands on your hips. This forces your shoulders-up and forces you to stand straight. Every time you stand, place your hands on your hips—make it a habit.
2. Learn to sit with your elbows on the table. This also forces your shoulders up and forces you to sit straight, with head-up—make it a habit as well.
3. Every morning as soon as you get up, and in the evening before you go to bed, face a mirror, raise your hands up your head as high as you can reach, your elbows as straight as you can make them. Keep your hands above your head and elbows straight until you slowly count to ten. Then rest your hands at your side

and repeat the exercise as many times as you can. Aim for 20 times. Eventually, aim for 60 times.

Canes and walking sticks. There are differences between canes and walking sticks. Canes are cut at the level of the low point of your arm swing. If your posture is stooped, a cane that is too low may exaggerate the curve, which in turn perpetuates your small, short steps. A walking stick, if it's the right height (shoulder level), forces you to walk straight. However, it's harder to learn how to properly use a walking stick than a cane, and your balance may not be as good as with a cane. Nevertheless, think of Moses: he used a walking stick, which forced him to walk straight—and yet it still took him 40 years to walk to the Promised Land. Had he used a cane it might have taken him 120 years! If your balance is good and you don't fall, then a walking stick may be for you. But if your balance is poor and you fall frequently, then a walking stick is not for you. Walking sticks can be found in many outdoor sports supply stores and they come in a wide variety of woods. Try using one that you like, or maybe different walking sticks for different occasions! Canes, too, come in more than just one variety. Adjust the height so you are comfortable. If you are having difficulty with balance, if you tend to fall, then a three-pronged cane may be for you. They are harder to use but give you more support and better traction. Remember, however, falls often occur when you turn. If you are in the habit of picking up your cane before you turn, the cane will not help—it must be touching the ground to support you! Learn to place your cane on the floor and use it for support *before* you turn.

Walkers. If maintaining your mobility requires more than a cane or walking stick, then you need a walker.

Some people are horrified by the idea of using a walker because the associate walkers with being an "invalid," but a walker is a device to keep you mobile—and if you're mobile, you're not an invalid, whatever physical challenges you may have. It is beats being stuck in a chair, or in bed—just ask anyone who *can't* use a walker which they'd prefer. A physical therapist or your doctor can advise on what type of walker will work best for you. The walker should be light but sturdy—light enough to transport, but sturdy enough so that when you turn, you don't first pick up your walker without thinking. If you do this, you will fall with the walker falling on top of you. Walkers with large wheels are easier to turn than walkers with small wheels. Walkers with ball bearings, especially the "U-Step" walker, may be even better. Remember to adjust your walker's height; if it is too low and forces you to bend, you will negate its benefits.

Wheelchairs. Wheelchairs come in a variety of types and can be very useful for trips outside the home. Most public museums, parks, movie theatres and concert halls are prepared to handle wheelchairs, and usually give folks in wheelchairs preferential treatment. Using a wheelchair will conserve your energy so you can better enjoy the event and the people who are with you. Mobilized wheelchairs are an even better way to get around and still maintain your independence. These devices come in many styles and colors. The batteries allow them to travel a long distance before recharging, and that can be as easy as just plugging it in to a wall outlet over night. They are expensive, but insurance may cover part, if not all, the cost. Second hand chairs that have been reconditioned may be a good value, too. Be sure to shop around and find one that is the right size and has the necessary features to be useful for you.

Think of your wheelchair as mounted infantry. Your wheelchair is the train, the truck, or the helicopter that takes you to where you need to go.

90. My partner has PD. We're both worn out. Should we take a vacation?

First, you need to decide what type of a vacation you want. Do you want to travel far? Go to a resort? Take a cruise? Enjoy nature? See an exotic part of the world? These are all possibilities. It may take a bit of extra planning, but you may be pleasantly surprised at the options that are available. Airlines make special efforts to accommodate people with disabilities. You just need to let them know ahead of time what kind of accommodation you need. If your destination is a particular resort or resort area, inquire whether the hotels have special facilities or can make accommodations to fit your requirements. Many cruise lines design cruises for people with disabilities and have medical staff on board to deal with any problems that might arise. Some travel agents specialize in arranging trips and vacations for people with special requirements. A helpful travel agent can find group tours planned especially for people with physical problems or pave the way for independent travel by helping you to connect with the services that you need to succeed. A travel agent can also find the right transportation, shuttles, and services to get you safely to the airport and assist you to get around in unfamiliar airports or make smooth transitions from one means of travel to another; a good agent will find the way to ensure safe arrival at your hotel or arrange appropriate transportation for sightseeing at your destination. The agent can even arrange to rent special equipment when you reach your destination or make the arrangements to transport your equipment with you. If you want to get away and see the world, don't let PD stop you!

91. Should I take a drug holiday?

If you're thinking vacation, don't think drug holiday: it's not a vacation. Before dopamine agonists were available as alternatives to L-dopa, and before Clozaril, Geodon, and Seroquel, were used to treat the psychiatric complications of L-dopa, drug holidays—temporary withdrawal of L-dopa to counteract side effects such as dyskinesia and psychosis—were the "rage." The holiday "purged" or "cleaned" the brain of excess L-dopa, but unfortunately it nearly did in the patient, as well.

The holiday was originally developed as a means of restoring the sensitivity of the dopamine receptors to L-dopa. In the 1970s many PD patients underwent what were called "drug holidays" or "L-dopa holidays" or "L-dopa drug holidays." The holidays lasted for several days to up to 2 weeks. Although many patients improved after the holiday, some dramatically, when L-dopa was restarted, the holiday was not a "holiday." As the symptoms of the underlying PD emerged after L-dopa was stopped, and the severity of the symptoms became apparent, patients and their families became severely anxious and depressed. Some patients became suicidal. Some developed difficulty swallowing, choking on and aspirating their food. And some developed an aspiration pneumonia. Some patients became so rigid they developed contractures of their feet. And some patients, because they were bed-bound, developed blood clots in the legs. Today, such "holidays" have been largely abandoned, replaced by a more skilled use of PD drugs, DBS, and, when needed, anti-psychosis drugs. "Holidays," if they are to be done, must be managed in a hospital by a neurologist trained in PD.

Two types of drug holidays were tried to treat L-dopa (Sinemet)-related problems. The first was the formal drug holiday, in which a patient was admitted to the hospital and Sinemet was withdrawn for at least 5 days or until dyskinesia disappeared or most of the mental changes clear. After the holiday Sinemet was reintroduced slowly. Follow-up studies indicated that after the holiday, some patients could be maintained on lower doses of Sinemet for several months. However, during the drug holiday, many patients exhibited a marked worsening of their PD. The worsening revealed their true PD state, the state they would have been in if they had not been treated with Sinemet. While patients were being withdrawn from Sinemet, physical therapy, respiratory therapy, psychiatric counseling, and nursing care became of paramount importance. Because holidays carry risk, today they are reserved for patients with psychosis for whom all other treatments have failed.

A variant of the drug holiday was the weekly 2-day holiday in which L-dopa (Sinemet) was reduced or stopped at home for 2 days each week. This was done in people who were experiencing mental changes, such as delusions, hallucinations, and agitation. The idea, unproven, was to "purge" or "clear" excess dopamine from the brain. A second variant of the drug holiday was the weekly 2-day in which L-dopa (Sinemet) was reduced or stopped at home for 2 days each week. The idea, again unproven, was to "desensitize" the dopamine receptors. This could be done safely in most patients, particularly if they were on a dopamine agonist during the 2 "off" days.

A rare but dangerous complication of the drug holiday was the "neuroleptic malignant syndrome." NMS is an unusual reaction to neuroleptic drugs (drugs such as Haldol, Stellazine, and Thorazine) and to abrupt withdrawal of L-dopa. NMS is characterized by high fever, severe rigidity, and ANS dysfunction. The symptoms of NMS may develop from a few days to a few weeks following neuroleptic drug use or a few days after abruptly stopping L-dopa (Sinemet). The muscle rigidity of NMS may be so severe as to result in immobility, which may lead to high fever, shortness of breath, decreased oxygen saturation, and death. The rigidity may also lead to massive muscle destruction with increased serum CPK (a muscle enzyme) and myoglobinuria (muscle breakdown products in the urine). The myoglobinuria may block the tubules in the kidneys, resulting in kidney failure. ANS dysfunction includes high fever, high blood pressure, and a rapid or irregular heart rate. NMS occurs in 1 percent of patients who receive neuroleptic drugs and is attributed by some to a dopamine receptor blockade in the basal ganglia and hypothalamus, and by others to a disturbance of calcium uptake in muscle. The mortality (death rate) associated with NMS, when not recognized and treated, is at least 20 percent. Treatment consists of the withdrawal of the neuroleptic drug (if this is the cause of the NMS) or the reinstitution of Sinemet (if its withdrawal is the cause of the NMS), supportive care, and the use of a dopamine agonist or dantrolene (a powerful muscle relaxant).

Making the Most of Life with PD

92. How can I become less anxious?

Anxiety is everywhere! All around us! And, if you have PD, you may be even more anxious. Anxiety, recognized or unrecognized, is an aggravating factor in many diseases, including PD. It's estimated that 95 million Americans, about one-third of us, are sufficiently anxious to seek help from our anxiety through counseling, meditation, alcohol, tobacco, and prescription drugs such as Ativan, Klonopin, Valium, Xanax, Paxil, and Zoloft. It's further estimated that 35 million people, about one-third of all anxious people, have **panic attacks**.

Panic attack

a sudden onset of panic with no apparent cause.

Situational Anxiety. Some, not all, anxiety is related to a particular event or situation and can be normal. Indeed, if during some events or in some situations you *weren't* anxious, if you *didn't* worry, *that* would be abnormal. If you *weren't* uncertain or fearful of hostile strangers, of flying in airplanes, of driving on darkened roads, of walking down dangerous streets, of being perched on dizzying heights, of encountering poisonous snakes or snarling dogs or speeding cars or unruly crowds, you might not survive! The critical question to ask is whether your anxiety, uncertainty, fear, or worry is proportionate or disproportionate to the event or situation. To determine if your anxiety is related more to external events (events outside your body) than internal events (events taking place inside in your body) answer the following:

Was your anxiety related to a
specific outside event or situation?   Yes   No

Describe the outside event or situation.

If you were an anxious, "high strung," or "stressed-out" person before you had PD, having PD will not calm you down; having PD is not helpful for stress management! But whether your anxiety is a psychological reaction to having PD or whether PD itself makes you anxious is an open question. PD affects regions of your brain that produce dopamine, noradrenalin, and serotonin—all chemicals that can decrease, increase, or modify anxiety. PD affects regions of your brain—the basal ganglia and the thalamus—that feed into what is called by some the "anxiety center of the brain:" the amygdala. The amygdala is an almond-shaped region (amygdala means almond in Latin) at the tip of each of your temporal lobes. The amygdala sits in front of a region called the hippocampus, which stores your memories—it is your memory bank. If you enter an anxiety-provoking place—a doctor's office, an operating room, a judge's chamber—as information about your surroundings registers on your eyes, your ears, and your other senses, and *before* the information registers on your conscious, thinking brain (your cerebral cortex), the information has registered in your amygdala. In the amygdala, the current information is compared with previous information stored in your hippocampus, your memory banks. As a result of this comparison (which might remind you of bad or unpleasant experiences in these places), you may become anxious even when there is no reason for you to be anxious: for instance, you may be entering a doctor's office to fix a phone, or you may be entering an operating room to change a light bulb, but because of painful or unpleasant past memories associated with a similar place, you feel anxious. It is possible that the sensitivity of your amygdala may change in PD and, as a result, you may be more anxious.

Anxiety in Parkinson Disease. Often people with PD experience anxiety in anticipation that their drugs are wearing off or they fear they are going to freeze or shake in an inopportune moment. But there may be more to it than an emotional response to an uncertain situation. The pathways that process this information pass through regions of the brain affected by PD. In studies of people with PD who have anxiety, psychological counseling helps in some, behavior modification helps in some, drugs help in some, and combinations of counseling, behavior modification and drugs help in other. What works may depend on whether the anxiety is related to a particular situation, or to a chemical imbalance in your brain, or to a combination of both—factors often difficult to separate.

Subjective or "Inner" Anxiety: At different times, different words are used to convey the feeling of anxiety. Words commonly used as synonyms for anxiety include *fear*, *uncertainty*, *worry*, *nervousness*, and *insecurity*. The words used to convey the feelings of anxiety vary from culture to culture and from language to language. Sometimes anxiety is expressed not in words but in physical symptoms. The symptoms that may accompany or substitute for anxiety include feeling dizzy, becoming flushed, feeling faint, experiencing a sensation of heat or cold that isn't related to an external physical source of temperature change, feeling jumpy, or experiencing involuntary twitching.

Objective, Physical or "Outer" Anxiety. Anxiety is translated into physical symptoms through your ANS. These symptoms are the basis of **panic**, defined as a heightened state of anxiety combined with physical changes in the ANS. At times of anger, fear, uncertainty, or worry, your heart can beat harder and faster, your blood vessels can narrow, your blood pressure can

Panic

a heightened state of anxiety combined with physical changes in the autonomic nervous system.

rise, your blood sugar can fall, your hands can shake or tremble, your legs can become wobbly, or your bladder and bowel can empty. Emotions of anxiety, fear, uncertainty, or worry combined with these physical changes can result in panic. The physical changes accompanying anxiety can be so powerful that a panic attack may mimic a heart attack. Because the ANS is affected by PD, PD patients may have less tolerance for anxiety, and panic attacks might be more easily triggered.

The Anxiety Questionnaire. To better understand anxiety and panic, you must measure it the way you measure fever or blood pressure. This is done through the Anxiety Questionnaire (Table 2) based on the Hamilton Anxiety Scale. Although the Anxiety Questionnaire has not been scientifically validated, in general, "Yes" answers to 15 or more questions indicate anxiety, which may be proportionate or disproportionate to the event or situation. "Yes" answers to 20 or more questions may indicate panic. To determine whether your anxiety is related to a particular event or situation, or whether it's related in part to your PD, take the quiz in Table 2.

Some of the conditions above may be symptoms of PD. Or they may be side effects of drugs you are taking. Or they may be related to anxiety. As you repeat the questionnaire at different times and in different situations, your scores may change. This questionnaire may be helpful in evaluating your progress or your response to counseling or treatment.

One factor thought to determine whether anxiety will turn into panic is your psychological makeup and your system of spiritual belief.

Table 2   Anxiety questionnaire

Below are common symptoms of anxiety. Some may also be symptoms of PD, or side effects of the drugs used to treat PD. Regardless, if you are experiencing a symptom, or have experienced a symptom in the past week, please select **Yes**; if not, select **No**. Record your number of "Yes" answers.

I feel my hands or feet tingling or burning.	Yes	No
I feel flushed.	Yes	No
I feel worried.	Yes	No
I feel unsteady or wobbly.	Yes	No
I feel nervous or irritable.	Yes	No
I feel my vision's blurred.	Yes	No
I feel anxious.	Yes	No
I feel dizzy or light-headed.	Yes	No
I feel fearful or afraid.	Yes	No
I feel I'm choking.	Yes	No
I feel uncertain.	Yes	No
I feel my hands or feet shaking or trembling.	Yes	No
I feel restless or jumpy.	Yes	No
I feel I can't concentrate.	Yes	No
I feel my heart pounding.	Yes	No
I feel insecure, I feel I'm losing control.	Yes	No
I feel short of breath.	Yes	No
I feel terrified.	Yes	No
I feel my stomach's upset or I feel nauseated.	Yes	No
I feel stressed or tense.	Yes	No
I feel faint.	Yes	No
I feel I'm sweating.	Yes	No
I feel panicked.	Yes	No
I feel my ears ringing or buzzing.	Yes	No
I feel hot or cold flashes.	Yes	No

"Spiritual Anxiety." Anxiety may arise when events or situations test your fundamental system of beliefs, a system that can vary from person to person. Was your anxiety, fear, uncertainty, worry related to a transgression of one or more of your fundamental beliefs? If you believe you transgressed one or more of your fundamental beliefs, which one(s)? A short questionnaire about beliefs or moral rules you may feel you've broken, modified from the Ten Commandments, appears below; by using this questionnaire (or a similar one you can create yourself if your belief system is founded upon different principles), you may get a more realistic assessment of whether your anxiety is based upon spiritual challenges.

1. You were faithful to your most fundamental belief   Yes   No

2. You did not let someone lead you away from your most fundamental belief.   Yes   No

3. You did not mock your most fundamental belief.   Yes   No

4. You used part of your day to do good deeds and charitable works.   Yes   No

5. You honor and help your mother, father, your elders, your teachers, and those who have helped you.   Yes   No

6. You did not harm anyone.   Yes   No

7. You did not commit adultery.   Yes   No

8. You did not steal.   Yes   No

9. You did not lie.   Yes   No

10. You did not desire that which is not yours.   Yes   No

Your anxiety was helped by (you can check more than one):

Counseling	Yes	No
Tai chi, or yoga	Yes	No
Exercise	Yes	No
Prayer	Yes	No
Prescription Drugs	Yes	No
Non-prescription drugs: alcohol, tobacco, herbs	Yes	No

Discuss the above with your spouse, caregiver, family, or friends, and discuss them with your physician. If you find that you are regularly breaking such fundamental rules, this might be a clue as to why your anxiety is not responding to treatment, and why your anxiety may turn into panic.

93. How do I apply for disability?

Many employers offer varying types of disability insurance as part of their benefits package to employees. If you are fortunate enough to be covered by such a policy, the human resources department of your employer will be able to guide you. There are also numerous other insurance policies for long-term disability, and if you have one, the insurance company should direct you as to how to apply. The one benefit that all Americans have paid into is Social Security, which, in addition to retirement assistance, also offers disability benefits. However, the government's definition of disability is very strict: the disability must last longer than 12 months, it must be "medically determined," and must prevent the person from doing any class of work, not just the type of work they were doing before the disability. There are two types of assistance available: Supplemental Security Income and Social Security Disability Insurance. The first, Supplemental Security Income (SSI), assists anyone with low income who meets the government's definition of disability. It has restrictions on income and assets, and the maximum benefit (at this time) is only $545 a month.

The second type of assistance, Social Security Disability Insurance (SSDI), is a type of insurance for which the applicant must qualify. To qualify, the applicant must be under the age of 65, have paid into Social Security for at least 20 of the last 40 calendar quarters, and his or her disability must have begun while he or she was paying into the fund. The amount of benefit the person may receive is calculated based on both earnings and the amounts paid into the insurance. At present time, the maximum benefit payable is $1,300 per month. There is also a mandatory five-month waiting period from the time the disability occurred before applying for this benefit. After age 65, the disability benefit will revert to retirement benefit, but the amount paid will remain the same.

Both benefits require an application submitted to the Social Security Administration. Once the Social Security Administration has verified all of the non-medical information, the application is sent on to Disability Determination Services (DDS), which will verify the medical aspects of the disability. It is a good idea to have copies of all medical records documenting your disability and submit them with the application. The

Making the Most of Life with PD

DDS will request any additional records they may need and may request an independent medical examination to verify the disability. The evaluation can take up to 145 days and may even be denied for lack of medical information. If it is denied, the decision must be appealed within 60 days and new medical information given to support it. No benefits are paid during the review or appeals process. If there is any question about the procedure or whether you are entitled to disability, it's best to consult with a disability lawyer.

If the claim is accepted, people receiving SSI are usually entitled to receive Medicaid benefits. However, Medicaid is administered by the state, and the payments are so low that many physicians will not accept them. If SSDI is awarded, there is a two-year wait to apply for Medicare. Medicare has two parts: one part covers hospitalization, including all in-patient care, and the second part covers medical doctors and outpatient expenses. The hospitalization part is covered by Social Security and costs the individual nothing. The second part, however, requires a monthly premium. Neither the hospitalization nor the medical expense policies cover the cost of prescription drugs.

While SSDI may be helpful, it obviously has some drawbacks. The long wait for approval before receiving benefits may be devastating; the two-year wait for hospitalization insurance could be a death sentence for someone with no other means of obtaining medical care. Prescription drugs for PD are very expensive and are not covered by Medicare. Although no one really plans to become disabled, perhaps the best advice is to take advantage of disability insurance while one is healthy so there will be at least some coverage while waiting for Social Security benefits to begin.

94. Are there services that can help my parents remain independent?

No one should have to give up living in his or her own home until it becomes an absolute necessity for safety or health reasons. If your mother has PD, and she is living alone, you must sit down and talk with her about her situation and what she needs to stay in her own home. There may be modifications that can be made to make it easier for her. For instance, if the house has an upstairs, then arrangements might be made for her to live downstairs, or if she must go upstairs, then a stair-lift might be installed. Making a shower more accessible so she doesn't have to step into a tub for bathing can also make a difference. Most communities do offer services for the elderly or people with disabilities. They range from special transportation to shopping or doctor's appointments to home health care or visiting homemakers. The services available in your mother's community can probably be found in the phone book, some phone books have separate sections that list the providers and their phone numbers and addresses. If your mother goes to a PD support group, they will be able to tell her what is available and who to call. Check with local chapters of national PD organizations to see what information they maintain on services in your area. Sometimes a county social worker can evaluate your mother's needs and make recommendations for services. Often, municipal and county services are stretched beyond their own limits and there may be waiting lists for their services. You could make your own arrangements to have someone come to help clean the house or maintain the yard or possibly have a friend of your mother come to visit her on a regular basis.

95. When do I look for a nursing home?

No one wants to go to a convalescent or nursing home, and no one wants to send his or her partner or parent to one. But there comes a time when it is impossible to lift and turn a PD patient, impossible to bathe or clean up after him or her, impossible to get a good night's sleep to prepare to do it all over again for another day, and even more impossible to care for him or her if the patient has developed dementia. Everyone has heard the "horror stories" about nursing home care, but living at home without proper care is a horror story, too. In a convalescent home, there are strong people to help bathe the patient, hot food and help to feed the patient, people to get the patient up out of bed and clean up behind him/her, and even social activities. And the care is given 24 hours a day, 7 days a week. So the decision to place a parent or partner in a nursing home must be seen as an opportunity to provide better care for the patient, to make his or her life a bit more comfortable.

Convalescent or nursing homes need to be chosen as carefully as choosing a neighborhood to live in or a school to attend. Locating the right one can be a challenge. As soon as you know that placing someone in a nursing home will be necessary, you need to begin planning. Your doctor or the hospital may be able to give you a list of homes, or you might turn to a national agency for long-term care and ask for their recommendations. Churches and fraternal organizations may also offer care. Visit several, interview the director, talk to the nurses, and observe the patients. Find out how many registered nurses are on staff, how many licensed practical nurses, and how many nurses' aides are employed, and whether they are permanent employees or are provided by a temporary agency. If the staff is from a temporary agency, they may not be as committed to the home as regular staff employees. Ask whether there is a social worker on staff and try to meet that person. Ask about the doctor on staff and find out if he/she will work with the patient's doctor, especially on the PD issues. Ask your own doctor about his/her recommendations for nursing homes and whether he knows the doctors at a particular home you're considering. Make a list of questions you feel are important regarding the care of your parent or partner and compare the answers from several nursing homes. Find out what services are covered and if there are any additional charges for some services that you may need to pay for. Find out about their charges and how to pay for their services. Consider carefully the financial implications for the patient and the family. Know as much as you possibly can before making a decision on which nursing home or care facility you choose.

96. How can I protect my assets?

Planning ahead for future care and establishing health care directives is a thoughtful consideration for your family. Having someone to talk to about it is important. When it comes to medical care, a living will can not only make your wishes known, but will guarantee that they will be followed. If you feel you may be unable to make decisions about future health care, you can create a durable power of attorney for health care (also known as a health care proxy) and designate a person you trust to make those decisions for you. A form for a living will can be obtained from a lawyer, a hospital, a stationery store or even off the Internet. Be sure it is properly filled out. You must sign the document in the presence of witnesses (which, depending on state laws, might need to be different people from the person named in the document), and some states also require that the signatures be notarized.

If taking care of financial matters is a concern, a durable power of attorney for finances can be useful. Again, check the requirements of your state for filing and registering these instruments. This instrument will allow you to appoint someone to handle paying your bills and managing your accounts while you are ill. It can give as broad or specific duties as you specify. However, the power granted in a durable power of attorney for finances ends at your death; the person you appointed will not be able to make arrangements for your funeral expenses. To do this requires a will. A will can be basic, no frills or it can be complex; it does not necessarily need to be prepared by a lawyer, but it may be helpful to have the advice of a lawyer if your estate or wishes are more complex. It does need to appoint an executor, whose job it is to make sure your instructions are carried out; it must be dated and signed by you in front of several witnesses who are not named in the will. Much more information on this topic is easily available, either on the Internet, in libraries, or from your attorney.

PART NINE

Hope

How long before a cure?

What are my chances of developing PD?

What can I do to help find a cure for PD?

More...

97. How long before a cure?

Before a cure for PD is found, its cause must be known. One problem in finding this cause for PD is that PD may not have a *single* cause; it could have *multiple* causes. There may be an environmental component, such as exposure to a toxic chemical, but the chemical may affect only those people that have a particular genetic predisposition. There may be an infectious component, exposure to some relatively "benign" virus that, in time, alters the genetic composition of your brain resulting in a loss of dopamine cells. It is important to note that at present no such virus has been identified, but the more we learn about viruses, the more humble we become as to what they can do.

Although the cause or causes of PD are unknown, much is known about how specific substances injure cells in the brain, including the dopamine cells. And, since the introduction of levodopa and the dopamine agonists, much has been learned about how the brain works. Drugs such as levodopa and the dopamine agonists Mirapex and Requip alleviate and improve PD. As more is learned about the brain, these approaches will be improved. Thus it has been learned that the early use of the dopamine agonists reduces and delays the appearance of symptoms such as wearing off or "peak dose dyskinesias." Newer, longer-acting agonists may have an even more dramatic effect. As discussed in Questions 30 and 42, PD cannot be cured, but its rate of progression may be slowed. Dopamine agonists such as Mirapex and Requip, discussed in Part 3 (Questions 23–30), and co-enzyme Q10 in doses of 1200 mg per day may slow the rate of progression of PD.

The Beginning. Parkinson disease (PD) was described by James Parkinson in 1817 at the start of the Industrial

Revolution. Is PD an outgrowth of the Industrial Revolution? Is it the result of a toxic by-product of the Industrial Revolution—one that poisons the internal environment of the brain? Or is PD a result of the increased lifespan that is itself a by-product of the Industrial Revolution? A perverse "bargain" where we live longer only to develop diseases not known in the past?

Genes and Lewy bodies. In 1913, a pathologist named Lewy discovered within certain nerve cells of people with PD, a round structure, or body, the Lewy body. Lewy correctly assumed the body was a marker, a tombstone, of cell death. In 1996, 83 years after Lewy, doctors found that Lewy bodies contain a protein called alpha-synuclein that is coded by a gene on Chromosome 4. They subsequently found that Lewy bodies contain at least two other proteins, parkin and ubiquitin, that are coded by other genes on other chromosomes. The genes are "blueprints," sets of instructions, that enable each cell to make the proteins it needs to carry on its specific activity. How genes are translated into proteins, how the proteins are assembled, how they're transported to where they're needed, and how they're removed after they've outlived their need, is under study. This will result in new insights into how cells live or die, and will offer us a chance to halt or cure PD.

MPTP, metals, and viruses. Drugs such as MPTP, metals such as manganese, brain injuries such as in boxing, and viruses such as those causing encephalitis, can cause brain cells to die, resulting in PD. But the dying cells do not contain Lewy bodies. Thus it's reasoned the process that kills them is different from that of PD. Whether you die from a bullet, an infection, or a poison, you're equally as dead; but in each case the process of dying is different. And so are the ways of preventing it. Lewy bodies may contain the secrets of PD, and their importance may transcend PD. In examining the brains of people after death, for each person with PD, there are 10 with Lewy bodies without PD. Are they at risk for PD? Presently PD affects 1 percent of all people age 60 years or older. If we live longer, will PD affect 10% of all people over age 60?

The Substantia nigra. In 1919, 102 years after Parkinson, and 6 years after Lewy, Tretiakoff, a pathologist, discovered a loss of pigmented nerve cells in a region of the brain called the substantia nigra. This is where PD starts. Lewy had "marked" the dying cells but he hadn't realized they were grouped together. Although the loss of pigment is obvious to the naked eye, and although many pathologists had studied PD, none had seen what Tretiakoff saw. There are 400,000 cells in the substantia nigra. They start to pigment after birth and are fully pigmented at age 18. The pigment is a normal product of cell metabolism. The pigment doesn't cause the cell to die, rather the loss of pigment is a marker of its impending death. The symptoms of PD follow the loss of cells. When you lose 240,000 cells, 60% of the cells in your substantia nigra, you develop symptoms. It's said that all of us (with or without PD) lose 2000 nigra cells each year. And, if we lived the Biblical "four score and forty years," or 120 years old, we would all have PD. At some point, and it's not known when or why, the cell loss accelerates: with perhaps 4,000 to as many as 10,000 or more nigra cells dying each year.

Discovering when PD starts, before 240,000 cells have died, and finding out why, will dramatically change our treatment approaches. The cells could die because of an inherited defect, a flaw in its blueprints. Or the cells could die because of an internally produced chemical, a naturally occurring free radical. Or the cells could die because of contact with an external chemical, an environmental toxin, one that breeched the cell's defenses. Depending on the cause, appropriate treatments could be devised to counteract it.

Parkinson–like diseases. PD-like diseases resemble PD and may, initially, be diagnosed as PD. Within 2 to 5 years, however, other features may appear that distinguish these diorders from PD. In most of the PD-like diseases the cell loss is not associated with Lewy bodies. There are several PD-like disorders:

- *Progressive Supranuclear Palsy.* For every 100 people with PD there are 2 to 5 people with PSP. On examination of the brain of PSP patients after death there are "plaques" and "tangles." Plaques are structures outside nerve cells that contain the protein amyloid, which encases many small blood vessels in the brain; this is the main finding in Alzheimer disease. Tangles are structures inside the cells, consisting of twisted strands of a protein called tau. Tangles are a principal finding in Alzheimer disease (in addition to plaques) and the main finding in a condition called Fronto-temporal dementia. But whereas PSP affects the same brain regions as PD, Alzheimer disease and Fronto-temporal dementia affects different regions. The relationship of plaques and tangles to Lewy bodies is being studied.
- *Multi-System Atrophy.* On examination of the brain after death the variants of MSA differ from PD by the regions involved and the absence of Lewy bodies. Moreover, MSA people has a distinct change in a type of cell, a support cell not a nerve cell.

- *PD and Alzheimer disease.* As PD worsens, nerve cells in other regions die. And, in advanced PD, Alzheimer-like changes take placs: plaques and tangles appear in addition to Lewy bodies. These changes occur in the substantia nigra and other regions of the brain. This is called Dementia with Lewy Bodies or Diffuse Lewy Body Disease. For each person with PD whose disease starts in the substantia nigra, there may be one person whose disease starts in the thinking part of the brain. This person is diagnosed as having dementia and not PD. The processes are probably the same, but the regions are affected differently. PD is like being hit in the arms and legs, and later perhaps being hit in the head. Dementia is like being hit in the head, and later, perhaps, being hit in the arms and legs.

- About 30% of people with PD eventually develop dementia. This is usually secondary to the changes of Dementia with Lewy Bodies. However, some people also have the changes associated with Alzheimer. About 30% of Alzheimer patients develop PD-like changes, while about 15 percent of people with PD have a family history of dementia. Whether this is Dementia with Lewy bodies, or Alzheimer, or both, is being studied. 15 percent of Alzheimer patients have a family history of PD.

Questions to be answered before there is a cure:

1. What's the "attraction" of PD for the pigmented cells of the substantia nigra? Not all pigmented cells are affected. Why some and not others?

2. What's the "attraction" of PD for cells in other regions?

3. Are Lewy bodies part of the PD "death" process? Or an attempt at repair? Should we stop them? Or encourage them?

4. In less than 1 percent of people with PD a gene causes PD. Three such genes are known. Are these unusual genes? Are there more than three?

5. The proteins alpha-synuclein, parkin, and ubiquitin, are clumped on Lewy bodies. Why?

6. Does a gene or a toxin trigger a process of "cell death?" Is cell death normal, nature's way of ridding the brain of extra or damaged cells? Or is cell death bad?

7. MPTP, manganese, brain injuries, and viruses can cause a PD-like disease. How relevant is this to PD?

8. How relevant are any of the PD-like diseases to PD?

9. Do people with PD who become demented have the same disease as demented people who develop PD?

10. Cells can be repaired by growth factors. Will growth factors lead to a cure?

11. Dying cells can be replaced by human stem cells. Stem cells may "cure" the slowness of PD but can they prevent or "cure" the dementia?

12. In PD there are problems with the mitochondria, the storage batteries of the cell. How important are these problems.

How long before a cure? I hope it comes about before the next edition of *100 Questions & Answers About Parkinson Disease* is published.

98. What are my chances of developing PD?

At this time these questions cannot be answered with certainty. One day, when we understand the genetics of PD, how the environment may affect PD, the cause (or causes) of PD, and how PD progresses, we'll answer these questions with certainty. Then, again, when we understand all of the above, we won't have to answer these questions because we'll have a cure.

Since we don't know what causes PD, we can only give approximate answers. To do so we state the following facts and make the following assumptions.

1. **Fact:** Your chances of developing PD increases as you grow older. In America, for all people, aged 20 to 70 years, the prevalence of PD is 35 people with PD for every 10,000 people. At age 60, the prevalence of PD is 100 people with PD for every 10,000 people. At age 70, the prevalence of PD is 200 people with PD for every 10,000 people.

2. **Fact:** In Iceland, where the entire population of 270,000 was surveyed, there were 572 people with PD. Family histories were available on all patients. If your brother or sister had PD, you were at least 6 times more likely to develop PD than if you had no family history of PD. If your mother or father had PD, you were almost 3 times more likely to develop PD than if you had not family history of PD.

1. **Assumption:** The facts about the chances of a brother or sister developing PD in Iceland is applicable to America. The facts about the chances of a

child developing PD if his mother or father had PD is Iceland is applicable to America.

2. **Assumption:** If there is no history of PD in your family, your chances of developing PD are the same as anyone else who has no history of PD in his or her family.

With the above facts and assumptions we address the following.

Question 1: I don't have PD. No one in my family has PD. What are my chances of getting PD?.

Answer 1: In your lifetime you have 35 chances in 10,000 of getting PD. If you are 60 years old you have 100 chances in 10,000 of getting PD. If you are 70 years old you have 200 chances in 10,000 of getting PD.

Question 2: I have PD. What are the chances of my husband (or wife) getting PD?

Answer 2: If you have PD, or your wife has PD, your wife's chances of getting PD (from you) or your chances of getting PD (from your wife) is NO higher than your getting PD if you have no family history of PD. In other words, PD is NOT "catching."

Question 3: I don't have PD. My father (or mother) has PD. What are my chances of getting PD?

I have PD. What are the chances of my children getting PD?

Answer 3: You are 3 times more likely to get PD if your mother or father has PD. And your children are 3 times more likely to get PD if you (or your wife) have PD.

Your chances of getting PD, or your children's chances, are 105 chances in 10,000.

If you are 60 years of age, your chances of getting PD, or your children's chances of getting PD when they are 60, are 300 chances in 10,000.

If you are 70 years of age your chances of getting PD, or your children's chances of getting PD when they are 70, are 600 chances in 10,000.

Question 4: I don't have PD. My brother (or sister) has PD. What are my chances (during my lifetime) of getting PD?

Answer 4: In your lifetime you are 6 times more likely to get PD. Your chances of getting PD are 210 chances in 10,000.

If you are 60 years of age your chances of getting PD are 600 chances in 10,000. If you are 70 years of age, your chances of getting PD are about 1200 chances in 10,000.

99. What can I do to help find a cure for PD?

Participation in clinical trials sponsored by drug companies offers both a very personal participation in research and the possibility of receiving effective, new treatments. This carries an element of risk and is not for everyone, nor is it even available for everyone. There are ongoing genetic studies of people with PD, which might help in locating a genetic marker. To find one of these studies, check the web pages of NIH. Since few people can participate in either clinical trials or other studies, the best participation is generous support for the non-profit agencies that help fund research. They are excellent candidates for memorial funds to remember a loved one who had PD. Gifts made to these agencies through estate planning helps fund the studies that will lead to a cure for PD. Another contribution you can make to become politically active: writing letters or making phone calls your representatives and senators. Let them know their votes are needed to support funding for research. Then encourage everyone you know to do the same!

One special and final contribution you can make is the donation of your brain (and other organs) to help scientists better understand PD. This requires advance directives from you and the cooperation of relatives who are willing to carry out these directives. There are four brain specimen banks; two that are supported by the National Institute of Neurological Disorders and Stroke (NINDS) and two private ones who also provide scientists with needed brain and nervous system tissues. Their addresses are in the Appendix.

100. Where can I get more information about PD?

This book cannot answer all questions you might have, so we have compiled a set of resources that will enable you to continue to find answers. The Appendix that follows contains a number of organizations, web sites, books, and other sources of information that are good sources of reliable information.

Hope

Organizations

National Parkinson Foundation
1501 N.W. 9th Avenue
Bob Hope Research Center
Miami, FL 33136–1494
E-mail: *mailbox@parkinson.org*
www.parkinson.org
Phone: 1–305–547–6666 (1–800–327–4545) (FL: 1–800–433–7022)
Fax: 1–305–243–4403

Parkinson Disease Foundation
710 West 168 Street
New York, NY 10032–9982
E-mail: *info@pdf.org*
www.parkinsons-foundation.org
Phone: 1–212–923–4700 (1–800–457–6676)
Fax: 1–212–923–4778

American Parkinson Disease Association
1250 Hyland Boulevard, Suite 4B
Staten Island, NY 10305–1946
E-mail: *apda@apdaparkinson.org*
www.apdaparkinson.org
Phone: 1–718–981–8001 (1–800–223–2732) (CA: 1–800–908–2732)
Fax: 1–718–981–4399

Michael J. Fox Foundation for Parkinson Research
Grand Central Station
P.O. Box 4777
New York, NY 10163
www.michaeljfox.org
Phone: 1–212–213–3525

Parkinson Action Network
300 North Lee Street, Suite 500
Alexandria, VA 22314
E-mail: *info@parkinsonaction.org*
Phone: 1–800–850–4726 or 1–703–518–8877 (CA:
   1–707–544–1994)
Fax: 1–703–518–0673

Parkinson Alliance
211 College Road East, 3rd Floor
Princeton, NJ 08540
E-mail: *admin@parkinsonalliance.net*
www.parkinsonalliance.net
Phone: 1–609–688–0870 (1–800–579–8440)
Fax: 1–609–688–0875

Parkinson Institute
1170 Morse Avenue
Sunnyvale, CA 94089–1605
E-mail: *outreach@parkinsonsinstitute.org*
www.parkinsonsinstitute.org
Phone: 1–408–734–2800 (1–800–786–2958)
Fax: 1–408–734–8522

Parkinson Resource Organization
74–090 El Paseo, Suite 102
Palm Desert, CA 92260–4135
E-mail: *info@parkinsonsresource.org*
http://www.parkinsonsresource.org
Phone: 1–760–773–5628 or 1–310–476–7030 (1–877–775–4111)
Fax: 1–760–773–9803

Worldwide Education & Awareness for Movement Disorders
204 West 84th Street
New York, NY 10024
E-mail: *wemove@wemove.org*
www.wemove.org
Phone: 1–800–437–MOV2 (6682) or 1–212–875–8312
Fax: 1–212–875–8389

Organ Donation

NINDS sponsored:

Dr. Wallace Tourtellote, Director
National Neurological Research Specimen Bank
VMAC (W127-A)-West Los Angeles
11301 Wilshire Boulevard
Los Angeles, CA 90073
(310) 268–3536

Francine M. Benes, M.D., Ph.D., Director
Harvard Brain Tissue Resource Center
McLean Hospital
115 Mill Street
Belmont, MA 02478
(800) BRAIN-BANK (800 272–4622)
(617) 855–2400
www.brainbank.mclean.org.8080

Privately sponsored:

National Disease Research Interchange (NDR)
1880 JFK Boulevard, 6th Floor
Philadelphia, PA 191103
(800) 222-NDRI (800 222–6374)
(215) 557–7361

University of Miami Brain Endowment Bank
Department of Neurology (D4–5)
1501 N. W. Ninth Avenue
Miami, FL 33101
(800) UM-BRAIN (800 862–7246)
(305) 243–6219

Publications and Information from National Institute of Neurological Disorders and Stroke (NINDS):
Parkinson Disease: Hope Through Research
An informational booklet on Parkinson Disease compiled by the NINDS.
La Enfermedad de Parkinson: Esperanza en la Investigacion

A Spanish-language public information booklet on Parkinson disease/Informacion de la Enfermedad de Parkinson.

Parkinson Disease Research Agenda
NINDS Parkinson Disease Research Agenda, March 2000.

Parkinson Disease Backgrounder
A backgrounder on Parkinson disease.

September 1999 Parkinson Testimony
NINDS Director's September 1999 Congressional testimony on National Institutes of Health Parkinson disease research.

Parkinson Disease: A Research Planning Workshop
Summary of a 1995 Parkinson disease research-planning workshop sponsored by the National Institutes of Health.

Researchers Find Genetic Links for Late-Onset Parkinson Disease
December 2001 news summary on recent findings in Parkinson disease genetics.

Parkinsonian Symptoms Decrease in Rats Given Stem Cell Transplants
January 2002 news summary on embryonic stem cells used in a mouse model for Parkinson disease.

Workshop Summary: Cognitive and Emotional Aspects of Parkinson Disease
Summary of workshop, "Cognitive and Emotional Aspects of Parkinson disease: Working Group Meeting," held January 25–26, 2001.

Third Annual Udall Centers of Excellence for Parkinson Disease Research Meeting
Summary of Third Annual Udall Centers for Parkinson Disease Research meeting. NINDS, the National Institute of Neurological Disorders and Stroke, is the leading supporter of biomedical research on the brain and nervous system.

Parkinson Disease Research Web
A National Institutes of Health disease specific web site to facilitate research on Parkinson Disease. NINDS is the leading supporter of biomedical research on the brain and nervous system.

2002 Parkinson Disease Testimony

NINDS opening statement to the Senate Committee on Appropriations, Subcommittee on Labor, Health and Human Services, Education, May 22, 2002.

Helpful Phone Numbers:

American Healthcare Association: 1–202–842–4444

Americans with Disabilities Act Regional and Technical Assistance Centers:

1–800–949–4232

The National Council On the Aging, Inc.: 1–202–479–1200

Elder care Information and Referral Services: 1–800–677–1116

National Council on Disability: 1–202–374–1234

American Red Cross: 1–800–435–7669

American Occupational Therapy Association: 1–301–652–2682

American Physical Therapy Association: 1–800–999–2782

American Massage Therapy Association: 1–847–864–0123

Health-Related Web Sites:

www.acurian.com (enrolling clinical trials, news and information on drugs in development, and Federal Drug Administration–approved treatments)

www.parkinsonscare.com (National Parkinson Foundation's caregiver Web site)

www.ahca.com (American Healthcare Association)

www.achoo.com (Achoo Health Director)

www.HealthAtoZ.com (search engine for health and medicine)

www.medhelp.org (MedHelp International)

www.caregiving.org (National Alliance for Caregiving)

www.globalrx.com (FDA-approved mail-order service)

www.geohealthweb.com (Geo Health Web)

www.caregiver911.com (Caregiver Survival Resources)

Helpful Videos:

The Educated Caregiver

A three-part videotape series dealing with care giving, a nice complement to *The Comfort of Home: An Illustrated Step-By-Step Guide for Caregivers.* To order, contact Life View Resources, Inc., P.O. Box 290787, Nashville, TX 37229–0787, or phone 1–800–395–5433.

The Parkinson Education Team
From the Young-Onset & Care Partner Support, Group Denver,
    CO. To order, contact Karl Ferguson at 1–303–830–1839 or e-
    mail *parrockies@aol.com.* Cost $20. Run time 1 hour and 25
    minutes.

8 Weeks to Optimal Health
Videotape companion to the book of same title by Andrew Weil,
    M.D. A holistic approach to better nutrition and improving
    the mind/body connection. At video stores or from *www.ama-
    zon.com.*

Tai Chi for Seniors
A 30-minute video introduction to the Chinese exercise form.
    Order by phone at 1–909–943–2021.

The Meaning of Health: Healing and the Mind
A PBS video production narrated by Bill Moyers. Order online
    from *www.amazon.com.*

Gentle Fitness
An award-winning videotape of six short routines to improve
    flexibility, balance, and breathing. Order from 732 Lake Shore
    Drive, Rhinelander, WI 54501, or order by phone at
    1–800–566–7780 (*www.gentlefitness.com*).

Sit and Be Fit
Videotape companion to the PBS exercise series. Special edition
    for PD. Phone orders: 1–509–448–9438 or Fax:
    1–509–448–5078 (*www.sitandbefit.com*).

**Catalogs featuring products to make living with Parkinson
disease easier:**
Sammons Preston: 1–800–323–5547

Sears–Home Health Service: 1–800–326–1750

J.C. Penney Easy Dressing Fashions: 1–800–222–6161

Adaptability: 1–800–243–9232

Caring Concepts: 1–800–500–0260

Glossary

Ablative procedures: procedures that remove damaged tissues through ablation, or destruction using heat sources.

Acetylcholine: a chemical that acts to transmit nerve impulses in the brain, the peripheral nerves, the heart, the gut, the bladder, and the muscles.

Akinetic-rigid syndromes: movement disorders marked by stiffness and a lack of movement.

Alzheimer's disease: a brain disorder characterized by memory loss and dementia. It is not related to Parkinson disease but has some similar symptoms.

Amantadine: a drug originally developed for flu symptoms that has been found to increase dopamine production and suppress acetylcholine in Parkinson patients.

Anemia: low red blood cell counts that result in fatigue and dizziness.

ANS: see Autonomic nervous system

Anticholinergics: drugs that block the activity of acetylcholine.

Antioxidants: substances that bind free radicals and prevent them from damaging cells.

Anxiety: a condition of fearfulness and stress that can exacerbate PD-related symptoms.

Aspiration: choking; accidentally inhaling food.

Ataxia: difficulty with walking and balancing.

Autonomic nervous system (ANS): the portion of the brain and nervous system that governs or regulates the body's internal environment.

Ballismus: a movement disorder that consists of sudden flinging of an arm or a leg.

Basal ganglia: a series of inter-connected regions of the brain including the striatum, globus pallidus, and thalamus.

Benign essential tremor: a common movement disorder related to anxiety. It is sometimes confused with PD because the principal symptom is shaky hands.

Biological marker: a specific protein or genetic change that distinguishes a particular disease or condition.

Bradykinesia: a primary symptom of PD that consists of slow movement, an incompleteness of movement, a difficulty in initiating movement, and an arrest of ongoing movement are associated with this slowness. Bradykinesia is the most prominent and usually the most disabling symptom of PD.

Bromocriptine: a dopamine agonist.

Carbidopa: a drug that is given with levodopa to reduce its side effects.

Cataracts: a condition in which the lens of the eye becomes cloudy and obscured, usually relieved with surgery.

Cerebellum: the coordinating center of the brain that acts as a "first responder" to information from the nervous system.

Cerebral cortex: the conscious, thinking brain.

Cholinergic receptors: enzymes in cells that attach to acetylcholine.

Chorea: movement disorders characterized by dance-like, flowing movements of arms or legs, often involving every part of the body. Also called dyskinesia.

Chromosomes: collections of genes that compose DNA. All people have 23 pairs of chromosomes in every cell.

Clinical trials: carefully monitored scientific studies of new drugs or treatments using human subjects.

Coenzyme: substances that are chemically related to other substances that have a specific effect. Coenzymes often are examined to determine if they can create similar effects to known enzymes without side effects.

Constipation: difficulty in passing stool.

Contralateral: on the opposite side.

Corpus striatum: an area of the brain named because of the large number of fibers that cross it—giving it a stripped or braided appearance (the name comes from the Latin "stripped-substance").

Corticobasilar degeneration: a movement disorder with rigidity symptoms similar to those of PD.

Deep brain stimulation: a treatment in which a probe or electrode is implanted and used to stimulate a clearly defined, abnormally discharging brain region to block the abnormal activity.

Delusions: a belief in something with no basis in reality.

Dementia: a loss of previously acquired thinking skills.

Depression: chronic feelings of sadness, despair, and helplessness.

Diabetes: a condition in which the body cannot process sugar, either because it lacks insulin or because the body has become resistant to insulin.

Diuretics: medications that help to rid the body of excess water.

Dopa decarboxylase: the enzyme that changes levodopa to dopamine.

Dopamine: a chemical messenger in the brain; loss of dopamine is a key factor in PD.

Dysarthria: difficulty forming or pronouncing words.

Dyskinesia: dance-like involuntary movements. Dyskinesia may involve the face, the tongue, the head and neck, the trunk, the arms and legs.

Dystonia: involuntary muscle spasms resulting in awkward and sustained postures, which may be painful. Dystonia can involve the eyes, neck, the trunk, and the limbs.

Encephalitis lethargica: the sleeping sickness that occurred early in the 20th century with some symptoms resembling PD.

Enteric nervous system: the nervous system that regulates the bowels.

Extremity: the endpoints of the limbs, e.g. the toes, feet, fingers and hands.

Facial mask: a symptom of PD in which the muscles of the face can no longer move, creating an expressionless, mask-like demeanor.

Free radicals: toxic molecules that arise from the breakdown and oxidation of foods and naturally occurring body chemicals.

Freezing: a PD symptom in which the person is unable to complete a

normal motion, such as moving a leg while walking.

Gene therapy: therapy that seeks to replace or repair a defective gene that causes a disease or condition.

Genes: long strands of four molecules that determine the way in which proteins are made. Genes are the basis of heredity.

Glaucoma: a disease of the eyes in which fluid accumulates behind the eye and presses on the optic nerves, in time leading to blindness.

Globus pallidus: a portion of the basal ganglia affected in PD. This region of the brain is known to be overactive in animal models of PD.

Half-life: a measure of the duration of the drug's action.

Hallucinations: a delusion in which a person sees or hears things or people that don't exist.

Hereditary: passed down through the genes from parents to children.

Hippocampus: the portion of the brain that stores memories.

Hyperkinetic: excessive movement.

Hypomimia: a mask-like expressionless face caused by rigidity of facial muscles.

Hypophonia: softness of voice stemming from rigidity in the muscles of the larynx and lungs.

Hypothalamus: a region in the brain that controls all the glands and the autonomic nervous system.

Impotence: inability to maintain an erection sufficient to complete sexual intercourse.

Incontinence: inability to hold one's urine or bowels.

L-dopa: *see* Levodopa.

Lee Silverman Voice Therapy: a method of training a person to strengthen his or her voice by singing loudly or shouting.

Lesion: a breakage or damaged area in tissue.

Levodopa: a drug used to treat PD that is transformed into dopamine by the substantia nigra.

Lewy bodies: small, iridescent pinkish spheres found in the dying nerve cells of people with PD.

Libido: desire for sex.

Magnetic resonance imaging (MRI): a technique that creates 3-dimensional images of body structures using strong magnetic fields.

Micrographia: a PD symptom in which the affected individual's handwriting becomes small and illegible due to decreasing control over hand muscles.

Mitochondria: cellular energy sources.

Motor exam: physical examination that checks a person's ability to move and respond to stimuli.

Movement disorder: any of a number of conditions that affect a person's ability to move normally, or that cause abnormal, involuntary movements.

MRI: *see* Magnetic resonance imaging

Multiple-system atrophy: a set of movement disorders with PD-like symptoms.

Muscarinic receptors: cholinergic receptors in the bladder.

Myoclonus: a movement disorder that consists of quick, jerking movements that can involve one finger or the entire body.

Neurologist: a physician specializing in diseases of the brain and nervous system.

Neuropathy: damage to the nerves in feet.

On time: in PD, the times in which a person is able to move normally without displaying symptoms of the disease.

On-off: in PD, the condition of alternating "on" (asymptomatic) periods with "off" periods in which symptoms such as freezing or dyskinesia are evident.

Ophthalmologist: a physician specializing in eye disorders.

Ophthalmoscope: a lighted tool for examining the eye.

Optic nerves: nerves that transmit sight.

Orthostatic hypotension: a condition in which the body's blood pressure regulating mechanism fails to respond adequately to abrupt changes, e.g. when a person experiences dizziness upon standing up.

Pallidotomy: a surgical procedure that can decrease dyskinesia, reduce tremor, and improve bradykinesia by interrupting the flow of neurochemicals from the globus pallidus.

Panic: a heightened state of anxiety combined with physical changes in the autonomic nervous system.

Panic attack: a sudden onset of panic with no apparent cause.

Paranoia: a belief that people are seeking to harm you.

Parkinsonism: a class of movement disorders with similar symptoms. Parkinson disease is one of these disorders.

Pergolide: a dopamine agonist.

Pesticides: chemicals toxic to insects that prey upon crops. Some pesticides are also harmful to humans.

PET scan: *see* Positron emission tomography.

Platelets: blood cells that cause clotting of blood and wound healing.

Positron emission tomography (PET): a scanning technique that allows the creation of 3-dimensional images of body structures, particularly the brain.

Postural instability: a lack of balance or unsteadiness while standing or changing positions.

Postural reflexes: reflexes that allow one to maintain balance.

Pramipexole: a dopamine agonist.

Presbyopia: a condition of the eye in which the length of the lens changes with age.

Progressive disorder: a condition that has progressively more severe symptoms over time.

Progressive supranuclear palsy: a movement disorder with symptoms similar to PD.

Psychosis: a mental disorder in which delusions and hallucinations are combined; the person is convinced that unreal things or people truly exist.

Pyridoxine: vitamin B–6.

Resting tremor: a trembling of the hands or feet that occurs only when not in motion.

Restless legs syndrome: an uncomfortable, aching sensation that is relieved if you constantly move your legs; usually occurs during sleep or while resting.

Retropulsion: the need to take steps backward in order to begin moving forward.

Romberg test: a test that observes whether a person asked to stand still sways backward or forward.

Ropinerole: a dopamine agonist.

Schizophrenia: a mental illness often characterized by auditory hallucinations.

Sebaceous glands: glands in the skin and scalp that secrete oil.

Seborrheic dermatitis: a scaling condition of the skin that occurs in PD patients.

Serotonin: a brain chemical that is related to anxiety and depression.

Sialorrhea: drooling.

Statins: supplements used to lower cholesterol that may also slow the progression of PD.

Stem cell: a primitive cell that has the ability to divide countless times and to give rise to specialized cells.

Substantia nigra: a portion of the brain with darkly pigmented cells that is a principal location affected by PD.

Subthalamic nucleus: an area of the brain located below the thalamus that acts as "brake" on the substantia nigra.

Thalamotomy: a surgical procedure targeting the thalamus designed to stop tremors.

Thalamus: portion of the brain that receives impulses from the nerves and transmits it to the conscious brain.

Tics: involuntary muscle twitches or movements.

Tremor: involuntary trembling, usually of the hands or head.

Urinary retention: inability to urinate even when the bladder is full.

Urodynamics: a series of tests that assess how well a patient can control his or her bladder.

Urologist: a physician who treats problems of the bladder and urinary tract.

Vestibular nucleus: a region of the brain stem that receives messages from the inner ears and eyes regarding balance.

Wearing off: a condition in which medications for PD slowly become less effective over time.

Index